SpringerBriefs in Applied Sciences and Technology

Computational Intelligence

Series Editor

Janusz Kacprzyk, Systems Research Institute, Polish Academy of Sciences, Warsaw, Poland

SpringerBriefs in Computational Intelligence are a series of slim high-quality publications encompassing the entire spectrum of Computational Intelligence. Featuring compact volumes of 50 to 125 pages (approximately 20,000-45,000 words), Briefs are shorter than a conventional book but longer than a journal article. Thus Briefs serve as timely, concise tools for students, researchers, and professionals.

More information about this subseries at http://www.springer.com/series/10618

Parikshit N. Mahalle · Sheetal S. Sonawane

Foundations of Data Science Based Healthcare Internet of Things

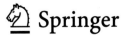 Springer

Parikshit N. Mahalle
Department of Computer Engineering
STES's, Smt. Kashibai Navale College
of Engineering
Pune, Maharashtra, India

Sheetal S. Sonawane
Department of Computer Engineering
SCTR's, Pune Institute of Computer
Technology
Pune, Maharashtra, India

ISSN 2191-530X   ISSN 2191-5318 (electronic)
SpringerBriefs in Applied Sciences and Technology
ISSN 2625-3704   ISSN 2625-3712 (electronic)
SpringerBriefs in Computational Intelligence
ISBN 978-981-33-6459-2   ISBN 978-981-33-6460-8 (eBook)
https://doi.org/10.1007/978-981-33-6460-8

This Springer imprint is published by the registered company Springer Nature Singapore Pte Ltd.
The registered company address is: 152 Beach Road, #21-01/04 Gateway East, Singapore 189721, Singapore

Preface

> *You are only entitled to the action, never to its fruits.*
>
> —*Bhagwad Gita*

Foundations of Data Science Based Healthcare Internet of Things book envisioned to present the precise and summarized contents that put more highlights on technological requirements, benefits and perspective use cases of integrating health care and Internet of things (IoT) and how data science can make better insights from these use cases. Since last decade, there is much advancement in very large-scale integration technology and semiconductor industry making electronic wearable devices cheaper and tiny. In addition to this, the Internet is also available at more faster and affordable cost as compared to the past. This has made the notion of IoT more adaptable and reachable to the common person. As one can see that, IoT is integrated in terms of many use cases in our daily life which includes smart home, smart office and smart factory to the smart city. When IoT was not known, the data was small and has become big due to the emergence of IoT only. As all IoT devices are connected to the Internet, the data has become big in terms of volume, variety, velocity and complexity. As the memory to store this data is getting cheaper and cheaper day by day, database management is not the problem today. However, the major concern is how to make sense out of this big data and draw meaningful insights?

This book focuses on how data science can enrich the application of IoT to the healthcare domain for making it smarter. In the first part of this book, IoT overview has been presented by referring to the standard definitions of IoT in the literature and new definition of the IoT is also discussed by considering various stakeholders and key enablers. IoT application phase in terms of the proposed 10C model is one of the key features presented in this book which will help IoT architect and developer to understand fundamental phases in application development. This book also discusses a layered perspective of IoT architecture so that it will be easy for the reader to understand different functionalities and IoT components concerning each layer. The concept of smart living is also introduced in this part of the book by referring to the emerging applications along with the technologies supporting smart living. Electronic health and mobile health are also presented and discussed in this part with different examples, and WHO guidelines are also referred in order to put forth the concepts more clearly. This part of the book finally concludes with the IoT design issues and challenges which are very important to design and develop IoT products and security solutions. The second part of the book presents application of IoT in healthcare domain for making human life easy. The need of converging healthcare IoT to the cloud and its benefits are presented and discussed in this part. Body area networks and their types like wearable, implants, wireless standards and technologies used are presented in this part. Remote patient monitoring and its potential advantages, electronic health records and its benefits are also discussed in second part of the book. Finally, second part of the books concludes with various healthcare projects, their design issues and implementation details.

The next part of the book deals with big data challenges in healthcare and data science techniques in detail. Due to digitalization of all clinical procedures and medical records, the data is available in structured as well as unstructured form. The electronic health records are mostly semi-structured format. The role of text analytics and natural language processing turns the data into value which is important to improve patient outcomes, streamline operations and manage regulatory compliance. Healthcare resources with data science tools and techniques are well explained in this part.

The main characteristics of this book are:

- A concise and summarized description of all the topics.
- Use case and scenarios-based descriptions.
- Ongoing and completed projects in the domain of data science, IoT and health care.
- Overview of healthcare tools and data set.
- Numerous examples, technical descriptions and real-world scenarios.
- Simple and easy language so that it can be useful to a wide range of stakeholders like a layman to educate users, villages to metros and national to global levels.

Data science and IoT are now fundamental courses to all undergraduate courses in computer science, computer engineering, information technology as well as electronics and telecommunication engineering. Because of this, this book is useful to all undergraduate students of these courses for project development and product design in data science and IoT. This book is also useful to a wider range of researchers and design engineers who are concerned with exploring data science for healthcare IoT. Essentially, this book is most useful to all entrepreneurs who are interested to start their start-ups in the field of data science, IoT and related product development. This book is useful for undergraduates, postgraduates, industry, researchers and research scholars in ICT, and we are sure that this book will be well received by all stakeholders.

Pune, India   Dr. Parikshit N. Mahalle
                                                                           Dr. Sheetal S. Sonawane

Acknowledgements

We would like to thank many people who encouraged and helped us in various ways throughout this book, namely our colleagues, friends and students. Special thanks to our family for their support and care.

We are thankful to Honourable Founder President of STES, Prof. M. N. Navale; Founder Secretary of STES, Dr. Mrs. S. M. Navale; Vice President (HR), Mr. Rohit M. Navale; Vice President (Admin), Ms. Rachana M. Navale; our Principal Dr. A. V. Deshpande; Vice Principal Dr. K. R. Borole; and Dr. K. N. Honwadkar for their constant encouragement and inexplicable support.

We are also thankful to Honourable Trustee of SCTR, Mr. R. S. Kothavale; Secretary Mr. Swastik Sirsikar, Dr. P. T. Kulkarni; Director PICT; and our in charge principal Dr. R. Sreemathy for their constant support and continuous encouragement.

We are also very much thankful to all our department colleagues at SKNCOE and PICT for their continued support, help and keeping us smiling all the time. We are very much thankful to our family members for their love, support and patience during writing of this book.

Last but not least, our acknowledgements would remain incomplete if we do not thank the team of Springer Nature who supported us throughout the development of this book. It has been a pleasure to work with the Springer Nature team, and we extend our special thanks to the entire team involved in the publication of this book.

Parikshit N. Mahalle
Sheetal S. Sonawane

Contents

About the Authors

Dr. Parikshit N. Mahalle obtained B.E. degree in Computer Engineering from Amravati University, M.E. degree from SPPU, Pune, and Ph.D. in specialization in Wireless Communication from Aalborg University, Denmark. He was Postdoc Researcher at CMI, Aalborg University, Copenhagen. Currently, he is working as Professor and Head in the Department of Computer Engineering at Smt. Kashibai Navale College of Engineering, and recognized as Ph.D. guide of SSPU Pune. He has 20 years of teaching and research experience. He is on the Research and Recognition Committee at several universities. He is a senior member IEEE and ACM, and a life member of CSI and ISTE. He is a reviewer, an editor of ACM, Springer and Elsevier Journals and a member of Editorial Review Board for IGI Global. He has published more than 150 publications with 1242 citations and h-index 14. He has edited 5 and authored 13 books and also has 7 patents to his credit. He has published a book on Data Analytics for COVID-19 Outbreak. He has delivered more than 100 lectures at national and international levels on IoT, Big Data and Digitization. He has worked as BOS-Chairman for Information Technology and is working as a member of BOS Computer Engineering SPPU and several other institutions. He has received "Best Faculty Award" by Sinhgad Institutes and Cognizant Technologies Solutions.

Dr. Sheetal S. Sonawane is Associate Professor in the Department of Computer Engineering at Pune Institute of Computer Technology (Pune) since 2003. She received Ph.D. from the College of Engineering at Pune University in 2018 under the guidance of Dr. Parag Kulkarni. She received Bachelors in Computer Engineering from Pune University in 2000 and 4th rank holder in Pune University for Master in Computer Engineering in the year 2006. Her main research interests are in the areas of data mining and information retrieval. She has published widely in international journals published by Springer and Inderscience and conference proceedings by IEEE and Springer having more than 400 citations. She is the recipient of Best Paper Award for her IEEE conference paper. She has also written book chapters in books like big data analytics by PHI Publication and "Semigraph and Their Applications" by Academy of Discrete Mathematics and Applications,

India. She is a reviewer of conferences and journals like Elsevier and Inderscience. She has more than 30 publications to her credit in international journals and conferences. In recent years, she has focused her research in machine learning, handling big unstructured data and graph model for representing and analyzing text document.

Chapter 1
Introduction

1.1 Internet of Things Overview

As stated by Mario Campolargo, European Commission, Belgium "Internet of Things (IoT) will boost the economy while improving our citizens' life". This indicates that an expansion of IoT services and products and application development will increase exponentially over coming years. IoT will play key role in smart living for every day-to-day activity. Mainly, IoT has become an integral part of every smart application which includes smart home, smart office, smart factory to smart city and smart country [1, 2]. There are many definitions of IoT available in the literature coined by leaders like European Commission, AutoID Labs, Cisco Systems and Tata Consultancy Services and are as follows [3, 4]:

> "From a network of interconnected computers to a network of interconnected objects", European Commission
> "The basic idea of the IoT is that virtually every physical thing in this world can also become a computer that is connected to the Internet", AutoID Labs
> "IoT is simply the point in time when more "things or objects" were connected to the Internet than people", Cisco Systems
> "A world-wide network of interconnected objects uniquely addressable, based on standard communication protocol" Tata Consultancy Services.

However, all the definitions have been formulated based on the business domain and revenue perspective of these individual organization or industries. There has been lot of debate on whether IoT is technology, framework, platform, architecture or all of these. Many information technology industries call IoT as technology because they want to generate business from this vertical. Fundamentally IoT is convergence of different embedded system components which include sensors, radio frequency identification (RFID) technology and smart devices in order to form proactive and smart service-oriented communication network. The main objective of this ubiquitous network is to provide seamless and context-aware services to all stakeholders

© The Author(s), under exclusive license to Springer Nature Singapore Pte Ltd. 2021
P. N. Mahalle and S. S. Sonawane, *Foundations of Data Science Based Healthcare
Internet of Things*, SpringerBriefs in Computational Intelligence,
https://doi.org/10.1007/978-981-33-6460-8_1

1

which includes users, devices, applications, Web services, etc., and the big data which is generated from all the connected device is posted on the cloud. The notion of IoT is now being transformed to new buzzword, i.e. Internet of Everything (IoE). The key concept of IoE is that all the devices surrounding to us can be connected to the Internet provided these devices have basic capabilities of sensing, computing and communication.

Consider the small use case of connecting Pen to the Internet. The first step is to add above-mentioned three basic functionalities to this device/object (Pen). First, we will add passive RFID tag to this Pen which has memory in Kb. We can store my employee id or any other identification number to this memory. Then, this tag is read by RFID reader which is Wi-Fi enabled and connected to the nearby access point. The identification number which is read by RFID reader is now accessible to access point. My laptop is connected to the Internet through this access point, and this is how my Pen is connected to the Internet. In the sequel, interconnection of such multiple devices results into the IoE.

IoT application development follows typical project development steps. In IoT, use cases are broadly classified as indoor use case (e.g. Smart Home) and outdoor use case (e.g. Smart City). It is very important to decide the category of the use case before design and implementation. Use case category helps to finalize the components required for application development, and in turn, it also helps to decide the cost estimation based on the type of components and quantity. In the sequel, establishing connectivity between the devices in order to establish communication is the next step. Once the communication between devices is initiated, then cooperative communication is started by involving multiple devices in the communication. When the devices are in indoor scenario, they are connected to the Internet through Wi-Fi, and when these devices are moving on the road side, they are connected to the Internet through 3G/4G LTE, WiMax, etc., leveraging convergence capabilities of these devices. After this stage, these devices which are connected to the Internet can generate contents (data) and post it on the cloud (remote storage on the Internet) or down the contents which are already stored on the cloud. These contents help to decide the context of use case depending on the type of data which is being generated. In addition to this, the complexity in processing and operations is associated with each step. This IoT application development process is depicted in Fig. 1.1.

Context and contextual information helps to impart intelligence and smartness in IoT use cases and applications. The basic objective of imparting intelligence is to make them proactive in the operations by replacing humans by machines. Data which is generated by several devices connected to the Internet plays key role in deciding the context. This data is referred as big data due to the main characteristics which includes variety, velocity, volume, veracity, value and complexity, and extracting meaningful insights from this big data is the main challenge. In big data life, the first step is to acquire the data, and then processing this data, next step is to perform analysis of this processed data and finally visualizing this data for better understanding. Different tools and technologies are required for performing each step in the big data life cycle. As stated in [5], RFID, IPV6, wireless sensor networks, M2M, smart phone, mobile Internet and semantics are considered as enabling technologies. Functionally,

Fig. 1.1 IoT application
development process

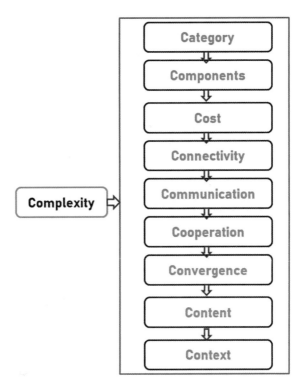

these technologies can be classified into categories. First group is the technologies require for acquiring context and contextual information, second group presents the set of technologies require to process this contextual information, and the last presents the set of technologies which are required to enhance security and privacy features of IoT applications. Smart healthcare, trading, smart traffic management, manufacturing, telecommunications, retail, logistics and social media are the major application areas where IoT and data science play important role. However, the main scope of this book is to explore various challenges, tools, techniques and how foundations of data science plays important role in healthcare IoT.

Researchers in the area of IoT and other allied fields have more opportunities as nothing is standardized so far in this field. In IoT, there are mainly three layers which include device layer (Layer 1) where all devices are connected, next layer is access network layer (Layer 2) where these devices use Wi-Fi or 3G/4G for establishing connection to the Internet, and last layer is application layer (Layer 3) where these devices are connected to the cloud and various services are deployed there. Unfortunately, protocols at all the layers of IoT are not yet standardized. The clear approach of using unique identifiers and name spaces for all types of devices (expedient and non-expedient) is still missing in the context of IoT. There is no confirming reference architecture for provisioning of IoT devices and protocols. There is further scope for the development of lightweight security and privacy protocols for resource constrained environment in IoT.

1.2 Smart Living

The adjective "smart" is connotation generally used to signify a work or a person which had done a given job in an innovative way by adding some intelligence and therefore also required comparatively lesser time for its completion. In similar way, one "single touch button" has made our human lives more comfortable, easier and most importantly time saving. "So isn't the life we leave in today's world should also be pronounced with an adjective 'smart'?". The answer is yes, the life we live with technology is actually a smart living. Smart living has become an integral part of day-to-day life. Offering improved contextual services utilizing the benefits from IoT components sensors, sensor nodes, RFID objects and smart phone is main objective of smart living. However, it does not mean that people who came before us were not leaving smart life. The every new innovation done in each era was part of smart life for the people of those eras. For example, innovations done for sending messages have started from letters, pigeons, telephones, mobile phones and now Internet. So in today's era, the Internet is smartest way to send messages, but we never know in future something more powerful than Internet may lead the world.

Big data analytics play key role by providing these smart services at lower cost [6, 7]. Smart living requires imparting proactive nature tidy appearance and intelligence in all applications making smart home, smart education, smart shopping, smart agriculture and smart healthcare. Home can be made smarter by providing functionalities like intelligent tracking of home user as well as visitors, remote monitoring and controlling of all home appliances, automatic placement of complaint if any home device needs repairing, proactive energy conservation by switching appliances off if not needed, making devices ON or OFF depending on the underlined context, etc. Tracking of old age people and assisting them for routine activity also require imparting smartness. The Government of India had announced to make India as Digital India, which includes the development of smart cities. And this smart city project includes six main components like smart people, smart mobility, smart environment, smart economy, smart governance and smart living. Thus, smart living in smart cities is indirectly a part of Digital India project. High level picture of smart living is depicted in Fig. 1.2.

- **Applications**

    There are various gadgets which lead to smart living and are listed below:

1. **Alexa**: The advertising tag line of the product, in itself explains the product usage. The line was, "To turn a house into home, you add love and to turn your home into voice-controlled smart home you add Alexa". The domotics provide house

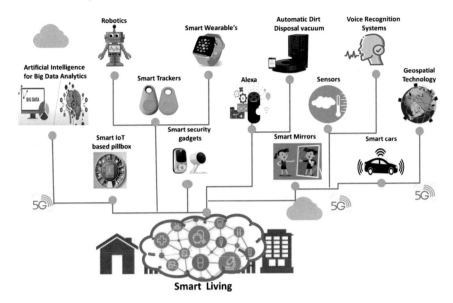

Fig. 1.2 Smart living

owners convenience, security, comfort and energy efficiency by allowing them to control all smart home appliances from their smart phones.

2. **Smart trackers**: Never lose your phone, key, wallet, pet or any other valuables by using smart trackers. These gadgets have a separation indicator which generates an alert on your smart phone as soon as your valuables are disconnected.

3. **Smart wearable's**: A smart wrist watch can show live heart parameters, whereas the smart sunglasses can capture videos and pictures in coordination with human eye movements. The mobility band for bind people is used to navigate by Toyota.

4. **Smart cars**: The driver-less cars is magic possible due to IoT and fifth generation wireless communication.

5. **Smart IoT-based pillbox**: A patient with dementia or any patient having too many medications generally has dependency on their caretakers. But the smart pillbox has made such patients life independent and easier, by scheduling reminders and tracking the pills. The smart pillbox has a separate compartment for each tablet. The infrared sensors in pillbox have an ability to send alarm to patients if it finds the compartment empty.

6. **Automatic dirt disposal vacuum**: The automatic dirt disposal vacuum not only dumps its own dirt but also communicates with a mop. This smart vacuum cleaner can locate the unclean surfaces with help of high-resolution cameras and then communicate these locations to mop for completing its job.

7. **Smart security gadgets**: These gadgets are more powerful and reliable than traditional security systems. They include smart doors, smart video doorbells having smart alarm systems which warn the owner to prevent their property from threats.

8. **Smart mirrors**: They are going to eliminate the need of changing rooms in shopping malls. As the consumers can directly have a live view of dress, they want to buy without even trying them on. The smart mirrors can also be used by drivers to see traffic conditions, blind spots, to see a satellite view for safe parking of cars and much other information.

After going through various examples, we can define smart living as, "Automation done in humans each daily chores may be at home, office or in public areas in order to reduce his work load and indirectly making his life more comfortable, easier, faster, precise, secured, time saving and stress free". Automation leads to smart living, which is turning the world into magical world.

- **Technologies supporting Smart Living**

  Prominent technologies supporting smart living are listed below:

1. **IoT**

IoT is the most essential and basic framework for implementing smart living. Without IoT, it is impossible to live a smart life. IoT can be said as an interconnecting thread among the things of IoT like smart devices, sensors and smart phone application.

2. **Sensors**

Sensors are core part of IoT system. Almost every device used for smart living has sensor that gathers and sends data to cloud. This interconnectivity forms base for IoT.

3. **Artificial Intelligence methods for Big Data Analytics**

The main key for automation is sensors, which collect huge amount of data in every single minute. Using big data analytics, the automation industry can build useful prediction models for smart living. For example, by using big data analytics in smart house environment, the smart device can also detect the abnormal behaviour of elderly people.

4. **Voice Recognition Systems**

Most of the smart devices used in smart living are hand-free means the devices are controlled by human voice. Therefore, a strong voice recognition system supporting multiple languages is also one of the basic needs of smart devices used for smart living.

5. **5G Communication Technology**

A smart living technology requires strong connectivity to work. The 5G connection will enable the IoT to work efficiently.

6. **Geospatial Technology**

The smart living applications rely on Global Positioning System (GPS) for connecting with remote users. For example, GPS is required to send a security alarms to an owner of smart house who is currently situated at remote location.

7. **Robotics**

Robotics is also a part of smart living. For example, kids robots used for teaching small kids or humanoid robotic translator used by outside visitors for Japanese communication in Tokyo.

1.3 Electronic-Health and Mobile-Health

Personalized healthcare is taking a good shape due to nuclear family culture, and old age people are staying away from their kids. Personalized healthcare helps to provide better healthcare and emergency services at lower cost. Remote patient monitoring is important activity in emerging smart healthcare which is enabled by embedded systems and body area networks (BAN) [8, 9]. BAN is equipped with patient to sense and monitor various physiological parameters, and these parameters produce electronic health records (EHR) [10]. Biomedical sensors are used in BAN for remote patient monitoring in smart healthcare which is enabling Electronic-Health (E-Health) and Mobile-Health (M-Health). Varieties of biomedical sensors are used for different diseases, and they have different electronic and embedded configuration. Biomedical sensors are mainly classified into four categories which include physical sensors (E.g. mechanical, thermal), chemical sensors (E.g. gas, photometric), bio-potential electrode (E.g. metal plate, microelectrode) and biosensors (E.g. enzyme, antigen) [8]. Heart and electrical movements in case of cardiac diseases can be detected with the help of smart wearable's (watches) and strap sensors, and these are mainly used in electro cardiology. Diabetes is another most prominent disease spreading at faster rate in all age groups, and it is very important to measure glucose level periodically in these patients. Tiny glucose sensing sensor or Google smart contact lenses are used for glucose level monitoring. Similarly, environmental sensors, GPS SmartSoles, motion detection sensors are used in the detection of diseases like asthma and Alzheimer.

Looking into the economics of scale and increasing complexities in the healthcare issues, storing and managing patient's history, information about their pathology test reports, routine medications and details about other complications is big challenge. The soft format of these details is referred as EHR. In the literature, there are various definitions available with different perspective and applications. From these definitions, it is clear that, ownership of HER is not with any single entity; however, it represents complete health details of the patient with any particular healthcare organization from the scratch. Basic functionalities provided by HER are storing and managing health information and data of the patients from the beginning, replication of the workflow along with effective interactions between various stakeholders (patients, physicians, notification and alert management through efficient decision support system), empowering patient by access to personalized healthcare details, processing and managing data available in various formats and providing support to various administrative tools.

- **E-Health**

EHR and allied technologies help to enhance E-Health and advancements in IoT are making E-Health operations more useful to the patients. E-Health follows compartment model [11] where the first compartment is patients which are located at their individual smart home and are equipped with BAN. BAN and associated biomedical sensors sense the physiological parameters of the patients periodically and continuously, and these parameters are aggregated at the home gateway of the respective smart home. This aggregated data is consolidated in EHR form which follows appropriated standards, coding system and frameworks. This data is from all home gateways is collected at the middleware which is second compartment of the model. This data collection is periodical or continuous depending on the patient classification and parameter classification. This is big data, and here, the role of data scientist plays important role by applying big data analysis, techniques and tools in order to produce meaningful insights. Healthcare service providers and physicians are connected to this middleware. The business logic is written at the middleware in order to generate alerts and notification to hospitals and physicians when physiological parameters of the patient go below or above thresholds based on the medical recommendations. Accordingly, appropriate action is initiated by healthcare organization either by recommending medications to caretakers or sending alerts to the relatives or providing emergency medical services to such patients. As EHR is most valuable asset of an individual [12], security and privacy of this big data at middleware are also equally important. Improved and lightweight security algorithms are required to protect this data when it is transmitted from first compartment to second compartment, when it is stored at the middleware and during access of this data from the third compartment.

- **M-Health**

The smartphone market is sky rocketing and the uses are multifold. Being in the ubiquitous world, availability of Internet at cheaper and faster rate due to advancement in broadband technology, all transactions and operations are being performed from mobile phones. Rapid advancement in mobile application development (Android, ios) has provided rich support for apps in all verticals. As stated above, the third compartment can be connected to middleware through various apps available for data access and alerts and notification exchange. Digital healthcare support through remote patient monitoring, delivery, recommendations and interventions are the key objectives of M-Health. HealthyYou Card [13] is one of most popular mobile apps provides search engine to search healthcare organization and also provides alert and notification regarding booking and cancellation. HealthyYou EHR [14] is another popular app which provides access to EHR. There is also support of artificial intelligence to support adaptation based on your working pattern. Another app to measure heart movements and electrical activity of heart is Zio Patch [15], and this app has also got official approval from food and drug department of USA. It provides uninterrupted monitoring with 100% assurance of authenticate and reliable data at lower cost. eWall for Active Long Living [16] was one of the most successful projects supported and funded by European Commission. The main objective of this project is to provide emergency medical services to old age people who are living alone and being cared by caretakers. This project integrated ICT technologies with IoT and BAN to improve on the active and healthy ageing of these senior citizens by applying artificial intelligence and big data analytics. Telemedicine is important area which is a result of IoT and existing technologies to provide medical support on mobile phones. Smart phones, tablets and wearable's are key enablers in telemedicine and M-Health.

1.4 IoT Design Issues and Challenges

As stated earlier, IoT is still in developing phase, and protocols, standards and algorithm in IoT context are not yet standardized. Essentially in healthcare IoT, preventive health, intervention, intelligent monitoring and critical disease management are the main issues. Some of the major issues while designing healthcare IoT are number of devices connected to the Internet particular time, scale of the devices generating content, entry points, decision points where the business logic is written, device classification, number of services, processes and convergence of healthcare IoT to cloud. However, these issues will vary from the requirements of healthcare organizations and their functioning. Life cycle of healthcare IoT devices mainly includes six functionalities [17] which are connection of the devices to IoT ecosystem, collection of the data (upload or download), correlation of data to context and contextual services, design of algorithm for calculation in order to make decisions, conclusion regarding ignoring or escalation of the events and establishing collaboration between patients and team from healthcare organization. In the view of this key design, issues and challenges are listed below:

1. **Network stability**

Provisioning of IoT devices and deployment of IoT application in unstable network where the connectivity of indoor Internet (i.e. Wi-Fi) and outdoor Internet (3G/4G) is risky and it results into unreliable services. Speed of source link, run-time detection of the quality of network and bandwidth, stability of the link across all compartment in healthcare IoT are important factors to deploy IoT products.

2. Energy management

Energy and battery capacity in IoT products varies based on the underlined use case. Mainly in healthcare IoT, availability of the IoT devices and services is more (i.e. downtime should be zero). In such cases, the sensors and actuators which are used in healthcare IoT should consume minimum energy, and there should be proper load balancing algorithms in place. Material science also plays important role in selection of the appropriate sensors from correct vendors, their configuration. Mitigation strategies in case of power failure, replacement strategies and software tuning are also equally important for better energy management.

3. Memory management

Run-time backup of critical data in case of sudden network failure is one of the daunting issues in healthcare IoT as once the time series data is lost, cannot be collected again. Selection of appropriate memory components and data structures (as memory is non-volatile in most cases) plays very important role. Designers should also consider the implementation of efficient decision-making algorithms in non-volatile memory and run-time creation of secondary partition in case of network failure.

4. Operating system issues

There is limited memory in most of the healthcare IoT devices (like BAN and biomedical sensors), selection of appropriate operating system (OS) (open source or licenced), size of OS and memory requirement, OS hardening, OS optimization are main design issues. Support of all OS specific device drivers, packages and libraries is also main responsibility of IoT product development team else there will be problems in provisioning and installation.

5. Data Management

Due to large number of tiny sensors and IoT devices collecting data from patients and connected to Internet, large amount of data is posted on the cloud. Therefore, there is extra overhead for data management and big data management in machine to machine communication towards healthcare IoT. Efficient data science tools, algorithms and techniques are required for better data management in IoT for drawing meaningful insights.

6. Performance and scaling

IoT products and application should not be designed by considering the scale (users and devices) of particular enterprise; however, these products should have capacity of expanding if the scale grows. During the period of expansion, the IoT ecosystem should be completely available without disturbing customer satisfaction (Trust Attacks) [18]. Expansion from design without much change management in

IoT application development process is main design issue in this context. Seamless expansion in scalability without affecting the performance is another design issues. In addition to this, IoT products should be designed to ensure performance metrics like latency, throughput, packet delivery ration, energy consumption, etc.

7. **Security**

As mentioned earlier, IoT use cases are divided into two main categories like indoor and outdoor, and each has their own design and security requirements. IoT applications and products being distributed and decentralized in nature, there are more security threats and are prone to attacks. Cyber-attacks on IoT devices and in turn exposure of crucial data are one of the daunting challenges in critical healthcare IoT. As stated earlier, in healthcare IoT, there is an exchange of valuable EHR between three compartments, and all these links need to be secured with lightweight security algorithms and techniques. Security by design and privacy by design are emerging techniques and suggest that the security measure has to be incorporated since the design phase. To design efficient solution, designers and developers should perform threat analysis and attack modelling of healthcare IoT is the first step to understand how exactly attack happens and which threat is responsible for this threat. The proposed security and privacy algorithms should be evaluated against known attacks by globally accepted test bed or security protocol verification tool before deployment.

8. **Interoperability**

The most of IoT products and applications are deployed on the existing legacy infrastructure and backbone is traditional wired network. Hence, backward and upward compatibility with the legacy networks in major design issue in healthcare IoT. Lack of interoperability creates problems like common application programming interfaces, failure in uploading and downloading information from devices using common interfaces, failure in securing the devices using third-party security solution and inaccurate controlling and management of IoT devices. To address this problem, defining standards, protocols and methods needs to be initiated.

References

1. Konomi, S. I., & Roussos, G. (Eds.). (2016). *Enriching urban spaces with ambient computing, the internet of things, and smart city design.* IGI Global.
2. Schaller, A., & Mueller, K. (2009). Motorola's experiences in designing the internet of things. *International Journal of Ambient Computing and Intelligence (IJACI), 1*(1), 75–85.
3. Mahalle, P. N., & Railkar, P. N. (2015). *Identity management for Internet of Things.* Wharton, TX, USA: River Publishers.
4. Mahalle, P. N. (2013). *Identity management framework for internet of things.* Ph.D. Dissertation, Aalborg University, Denmark.
5. Mahalle, P. N., & Dhotre, P. S. (2019). *Context-aware pervasive systems and applications.* https://www.springer.com/gp/book/9789813299511.

6. Bhatt, C., Dey, N., & Ashour, A. S. (Eds.). (2017). Internet of things and big data technologies for next generation healthcare.

7. Dey, N., Hassanien, A. E., Bhatt, C., Ashour, A., & Satapathy, S. C. (Eds.). (2018). *Internet of things and big data analytics toward next-generation intelligence* (pp. 3–549). Berlin: Springer.

8. Elhayatmy, G., Dey, N., & Ashour, A. S. (2018). Internet of things based wireless body area network in healthcare. In *Internet of things and big data analytics toward next-generation intelligence* (pp. 3–20). Cham: Springer.

9. How wearable heart-rate monitors work, and which is best for you. https://arstechnica.com/gad gets/2017/04/how-wearable-heart-rate-monitors-work-and-which-is-best-for-you/. Accessed 28 Dec 2017.

10. Sinha, P. K., Sunder, G., Bendale, P., Mantri, M., & Dande, A. (2012). *Electronic health record: Standards, coding systems, frameworks, and infrastructures*. Wiley. https://doi.org/10.1002/9781118479612. Print ISBN 9781118281345, Online ISBN 9781118479612.

11. Mahalle, P. N., & Shinde, G. R. (2020). OAuth-based authorization and delegation in smart home for the elderly using decentralized identifiers and verifiable credentials. In *Security issues and privacy threats in smart ubiquitous computing*. Singapore: Springer Nature.

12. McKeeby, J. W., & Coffey, P. S. (2018). The importance and use of electronic health records in clinical research. In: J. I. Gallin, F. P. Ognibene, & L. L. Johnson (Eds.), *Principles and practice of clinical research* (4th ed., pp. 687–702). Academic Press. ISBN 9780128499054.

13. https://healthyyoucard.com/.

14. https://play.google.com/store/apps/details?id=in.mediit.android.healthyyoudoctor&hl=en_IN.

15. Tung, C. E., Su, D., Turakhia, M. P., & Lansberg, M. G. (2015). Diagnostic yield of extended cardiac patch monitoring in patients with stroke or TIA. *Frontiers in Neurology, 5,* 266.

16. https://cordis.europa.eu/project/id/610658.

17. Lake, D., Milito, R., Morrow, M., & Vargheese, R. (2014). Internet of things: architectural framework for ehealth security. *Journal of ICT Standardization, 1.*

18. Mahalle, P. N., & Shinde, G. R. (2020). Trust attacks in internet of things: A new data-centric cybercrime on enterprise use case. In *Proceedings of 2nd International Conference on Advanced Computing Technologies and Applications*. Springer.

Chapter 2
Internet of Things in Healthcare

2.1 Introduction

Extending IoT for healthcare domain creates lot of opportunities to improve the lifestyle of the people by replacing traditional healthcare system by smart healthcare system. The current healthcare system works on detect and treat; however, the smart healthcare system follows the methodology of prevention by proactive monitoring and if required treat by remote patient monitoring. The way data is stored and accessed to deliver intelligent seamless services to the patients, tools and techniques designed to provide proactive monitoring, mechanism to support prevention mechanism than detection mechanism enables smart preventive healthcare [1]. Fortunately, the vision and mission of healthcare IoT is supported by all the countries globally, and the budget provision is also made available by these countries [2]. Considering the recent example of Covid-19 pandemic [3], US Health Ministry has also revised the budget for applying healthcare IoT to any pandemic [4]. This also indicates that in the coming years, there are more opportunities for investors, manufacturer, healthcare organization and healthcare IoT product designers and developers to invest more to generate better revenue.

In small standalone consumer applications like the smart home and care for disabled and elders, the requirement for capabilities such as processing power, storage space and computing can be facilitated by the participating devices (mobile phones, Raspberry Pi kits, etc.) themselves. The resource requirements for such applications are lesser. However, for larger commercial real-time applications such as healthcare, transportation, etc., the demand for resources is huge due to the enormous data that is collected and also the complexity of computations that are involved in the system. The demand for resources (storage, servers and processors) in such huge applications many a times cannot be satisfied by the participating devices alone. This is where cloud comes in handy by catering to larger business needs.

© The Author(s), under exclusive license to Springer Nature Singapore Pte Ltd. 2021
P. N. Mahalle and S. S. Sonawane, *Foundations of Data Science Based Healthcare Internet of Things*, SpringerBriefs in Computational Intelligence,
https://doi.org/10.1007/978-981-33-6460-8_2

IoT cloud convergence for healthcare IoT is a need of today. The key services provided by the cloud like processing, computation, dynamic provisioning and virtualization in IoT application play very important role in the healthcare domain. There are potential cloud platform service providers available in the market (Eg. Google, IBM, AMAZON, Microsoft), and comparative study of these platforms is very important so that users can utilize the benefits of underlined applications. There are more opportunities to design and develop IoT cloud convergence architecture so that enhanced services with better performance can be extended to the users. There are also various test beds which need to be explored [5] for research and development purposes. Smart computing aspects (advanced) for smart healthcare are important and need of the hour technologies in today's connected and demanding world. The emerging technology for smart computing after machine learning and deep learning [6] is cognitive computing [7]. It is available in the market in the form of various platform and tool like Deep Mind, Watson, etc. Commonly used algorithms, tools, techniques along with potential case studies are also important in order to apply cognitive computing in smart healthcare.

Smart computing in the context of IoT cloud depicts the introduction of advanced computing capabilities including real-time awareness of the surrounding environment and analytics (of the big data detected from various sensors and devices) into the IoT applications by leveraging the capabilities of cloud. This enables incorporating intelligence into the decision-making process with the advanced resources made available through the cloud. The revolution in different technologies like cloud computing, IoT, cognitive computing, big data analytics and deep learning has made smart application and efficient services with less human intervention. This convergence of different technologies, especially, cloud computing has become skyrocketing and eventually leads to many personal and business opportunities.

2.2 Body Area Networks

Due to rapid advancement in very large-scale integration, semiconductor technology and wireless communication, it is possible to manufacture low-power and intelligent tiny sensor nodes. These sensor nodes can be placed around human body for the monitoring purpose producing body area networks (BAN). IEEE 802.15.6 [8] is a standard which is specifically used for reliable low-power short-range wireless communication, and this standard is used in BAN for reliable communication around human body. These sensor nodes designed and manufactured in such a way that they do not have any adverse and negative impact on the human body. BAN is also used in applications like military, sports, mechatronics industries, research due to minimum power consumption. The main characteristics of BAN include cost effective, energy efficient, reliable and also support heterogeneity which is the main requirement for healthcare IoT [9]. For optimizing power consumption and cost, another emerging low-power wireless personal area network standard is Bluetooth for Low Energy (BLE), and the stable version is BLE 4.0 [10]. BLE 4.0 enables

Table 2.1 BLE 4.0 factsheet

S. No.	Parameter	Details
1	Range	150 m
2	Output power	10 mW
3	Maximum current	15 mA
4	Latency	3 ms
5	Topology	Star
6	Connection	> 2 billion
7	Modulation	GFSK@2.4 GHz
8	Robustness	Adaptive Frequency Hoping, 24 bit CRC
9	Security	128 bit AES CCM
10	Sleep current	1 μA
11	Modes	Broadcast, Connection, Event Data Models Reads, Writes

wireless device to device connectivity with low power consumption as compared with earlier versions. The main feature of BLE 4.0 is devices remain connected, and pairing does not get disturbed even there is no data transfer active between the devices. Due to these features, BLE 4.0 plays vital role in design and development of BAN (like wearable computing devices, monitoring devices, etc.). Throughput is not significant performance metrics for BLE 4.0 as it not designed for streaming. BLE 4.0 supports data rate of 1Mbps; however, it is not suitable for applications which include file transfer. IoT applications require the data exchange between the devices and Web services, and BLE 4.0 also provides technologies to connect IoT devices and services running on Web. BLE 4.0 also supports IP addresses. Table 2.1 presents the factsheet of BLE 4.0.

BAN and associated devices are connected to Internet for data exchange and also interoperable with other wireless standards like wireless sensor networks, Bluetooth, ZigBee and Wi-Fi. BAN covers variety of applications and is broadly divided into two categories like medical applications and non-medical applications. Medical application includes wearable BAN and is used in monitoring fatigue and battle readiness of on-field soldiers, intelligent sport training, monitoring of asthma and wearable health monitoring. Medial applications of BAN are further classified into following three categories and described below

a. **Wearable BAN**

This category includes use of cameras, biomedical sensors integrated with wireless networks to enable monitoring and notification management. Monitoring of drivers drowsiness, fatigue identification of the soldier on field, sleep tagging, wearable health monitoring are some prominent use cases of this category. Wearable BAN also plays key role in rehabilitation of impaired as well as disabled people by extending sensing capabilities. There is also need of energy-efficient wearable BAN architectures in order to get real-time and more accurate data at lower cost. Security and privacy issues are equally important as there is exchange of sensitive information between the devices and Internet.

b. **Implant BAN**

In implant BAN, micro devices are placed in the human body under skin or in the blood for monitoring various physiological parameters. Implant BAN can be operated with the help of technical persons and medical experts. Biomedical sensors are placed in the body for continuous monitoring of glucose level in diabetic patients. This mechanism works as a preventive mechanism, and human life can be saved from future consequences. Heart rate monitoring in cardiovascular disease is another interesting use case where heart rate and other episodic events are continuously monitored using BAN, and cardiac arrest as well as heart attacks can be prevented by placing BAN device in human body. Critical and emergency healthcare prevention can be effectively done with the help of implant BAN.

c. **Remote Control of Medical Devices**

Due to ubiquitous computing and performing action in anytime, anything, anywhere manner, the concept of ambient-assisted living, telemedicine and remote patient monitoring is coming up. In case of chronic diseases, controlling BAN devices remotely for monitoring purpose helps to prevent reoccurring of the disease. Symptoms and change in the controlling parameters can be detected to appropriate medication, and drug can be administered. Telemedicine is useful for the patients living in rural area which enables remote monitoring of vital biological parameters remotely through wireless medium. Telemedicine provides good interface between patient and healthcare organization. Telemedicine also provides better guidance to the physicians when patient is in transit from village to the city hospital in emergency.

802.15.6 standard for BAN supports only two layers, i.e. physical layer (PHY) and medium access control (MAC) layer. Network layer, transport layer and other layers are supported by this standard. However, these layers are designed by third-party vendors and integrated with the existing standard. These two layers are designed to support low-power, optimized cost and short-range reliable wireless communication. Sending and receiving of data, radio activation and deactivation, assessment of channel and these functionalities and design issues vary depending on whether the application is medical or non-medical. There are three different physical layers in 802.15.6 standards which are human body communication, narrow band and ultrawide band [11], and one of the layers is used depending on the underline applications. Channel access is coordinated and controlled by MAC layer which is built on the top of PHY layer. The coordinator is responsible for channelling and frame management, and there are three access modes which are beacon mode, non-beacon mode (super frame boundaries) and non-beacon mode (without super frame boundaries). As BAN is used in mostly healthcare applications, availability of devices associated with BAN is very crucial issue as there is a need of continuous monitoring of vital parameters. There can be attack on availability causing delay or blocking for monitoring, and it can create problem to the patient life. There should be also backup provision to replace entire functioning on the alternative devices to avoid downtime. Trust management is another daunting issue in BAN because there should be trusted communication as well as trusted communication link between BAN and health-care organization. There should be lightweight trust management solution in place. Intelligent mechanism to calculate trust score between communicating devices in BAN requires more attention. Mutual identity establishment to verify the identity of devices or entities on both sides is also important to confirm legitimate devices. Selective disclosure, authorization and access control solution also require more attention. There are emerging frameworks like OAUTH [12, 13], UMA 2.0 [14, 15] also need to be revisited to ensure that how these frameworks can be used in smart healthcare domain. Better authorization processes can be utilized through these frameworks to prevent medical errors for accurate healthcare services. Patient empowerment by giving more controlling right on their personal data is also main objective of these frameworks.

Human body absorption causes much path loss, and there is a need to control this path loss. This path loss needs to be controlled using different types of multihop links as well as sensors at different location across transmission link. Environmental conditions also affect the performance of BAN which includes incomplete data transmission, data transmission with errors, sensor failure, link failure as well as issues caused due to interference. Design of energy-efficient, tiny and non-invasive biomedical sensors is main requirement for manufacturers. Signal processing of information collected from various sensory resources can be useful to avoid data rate on the internal network. For this purpose, there is a requirement of load balancing between data processing at devices and data transfer bin in the network. Designers should also consider the achievement of quality of service parameters, power source and conservation at various layers in BAN because BAN channels are heavily attenuated by human body.

2.3 Remote Patient Monitoring

Due to advancement in information technology tools, techniques and programming support as well as Internet availability, connectivity of user to user, user to device, device to user and device to device has become faster and easy. This enables remote patient monitoring (RPM) more efficient and thus making growing market for smart healthcare. In healthcare domain, day by day the severity of diseases is increasing at faster rate, and new pandemic diseases like Covid-19 [16] are arriving suddenly affecting human lives and global economy. Observation-based diagnosis and treatment is becoming absolute now due to the disease severity, and now, physiological parameters centric is evolving where all diagnosis and treatment is carried out based on the values of these parameters. In the sequel, there is need to monitor these biological parameters like heart rate, blood pressure, glucose level, pulse rate, electrical signal flow in the brain, etc., continuously or periodically. RPM enables more precise and immediate run-time decision by electronically monitoring these parameters. RPM is defined as below:

> Remote patient monitoring is proactive collection of physiological parameters of the patients through BAN either periodically or continuously for initiating accurate decisions and also managing the deployment of life support devices.

Essentially, RPM is required for few categories of the patients which include patients having regular illness problems due to any of the disease (like disease related to heart, lungs, lever, brain, etc.), the patients which are supposed to face major health problem due to any disease in near future, patients who are at high risk due to critical health conditions due to any organ damage, the patients which are already in intensive care units due to multiple severity conditions of many diseases, and last is the special category of mother and baby during delivery.

As stated earlier, in RPM, there are three vertical layers. The first layer is BAN, second layer is middleware which can be home gateway or medical gateway, and the third layer is application layer where all medical services are running to which all physicians and healthcare organizations are connected. The high-level view of RPM is depicted in Fig. 2.1. There is a smart home equipped with smart devices like fan, water metre, electricity metre, temperature sensor, smoke sensor and patients among house owners if any equipped with BANs. The patients are continuously/periodically monitored through biomedical sensors, and the values of different physiological parameters are collected at gateway through local wireless connectivity (Zigbee, Bluetooth, WPAN). These patient details in the form of EHR are then transmitted to the middleware (MW) through the Internet which is central repository managed and maintained by either healthcare organization or trusted third-party IT service providers. At his MW, the business logic is written for real-time consent, resource

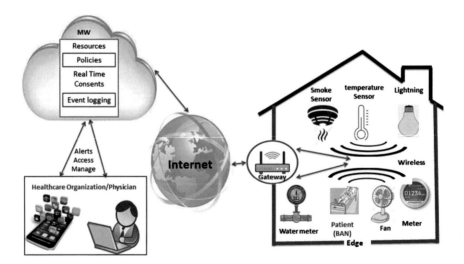

Fig. 2.1 High-level view of RPM

management, event logging and policies are also written in order to perform authorization access control. Based on the conditions and threshold values of different parameters taken into consideration in business logic, alerts and notifications are generated to the healthcare organizations or physicians. Potential advantages of the RPM are listed below:

1. **Improved collaboration between patients and healthcare organization**
   RMP enables active participation of patients during their interaction with the healthcare organization, and thus, it improves collaboration between patient and healthcare organizations (doctor, physicians, etc.).

2. **Better utilization of resources**
   Due to RMP, the patients can be diagnosed remotely, and decision can be taken whether the patients' needs to be admitted physically to the hospital or not. This results into optimized utilization of the resources, and also, it reduces the work load of paramedical staff.

3. **Enhanced care for chronic diseases**
   With the rich data set collected from various patients suffering from chronic diseases, their management and care can be enhanced by applying data science techniques to these data sets with the help of resulted meaningful insights.

4. **Increased patient accountability**
   As the patients are aware that their EHR is being exchanged and shared with healthcare organization through RPM, it gives patients assurance about their care, and thus, it increases the patient accountability.

5. **Improved quality of care**
   Run-time time accurate decisions, precise diagnosis, real-time data analytics, recommendations and preventive measures through RPM help to improve the quality of care of patients.

Design and Implementation

There are multiple ways to design RPM system based on the requirements, and design issues vary from one healthcare organization to other. The basic hardware components require is any RPM system is i) microcontroller for analog signal interface, ii)GSM module, iii)various biomedical sensors, iv)smart phones for interfacing and communication and v) protocols like Zigbee, Bluetooth or WPAN for local connectivity. There is also central patient monitoring system associated with every RPM which is configured on computer with adequate resources. For any RPM, data collection, data processing and data delivery are three main functionalities which are described below:

- Data acquisition
  Sensor and embedded devices are involved in data acquisition. These devices use BAN or WPAN for collecting data from multiple sources and then aggregated at the gateway. Sensors are used in two modes contactless mode and with contact methods [17] where in contactless methods, sensors do not touch the human body.

- Data processing
  Data processing requires computing infrastructure for data reception, transmission and data processing. This processing can be carried out at the terminal or gateway available at the hospital with required computing resources, or it can also be carried out at the smart phone of the doctor. This processing task also can be made context-aware, and the location can be decided at the run-time depending on the run-time load of either gateway or smart phone of the doctor.
- Data delivery
  The underline communication infrastructure uses appropriate communication protocol in order to connect data acquisition system to data processing system, and the data is delivered to healthcare organization or doctor as and when required on demand.
  The main challenges for the designers are to decide on the method of connecting biomedical sensors to the human body (with contact or contactless), the type and configuration of the sensors, choice of different big data processing algorithms and their implementations as well as communication protocol to be used for connecting the three modules like data acquisition, data processing and data delivery. Some RPM, design issues and technologies required can be referred in [18, 19].

2.4 Electronic Health Record

As mentioned in the Chap. 1, the main objective of electronic health record (EHR) is to transform existing paper-based system to the paper less system by converting hard data into soft form. Use of ICT-based tools and techniques enable easy and centralized access to this soft data in ubiquitous manner. EHR can be easily transferred from one location to another location electronically faster due to availability of Internet at faster rate. Extending smart healthcare has become more reliable, coordinated and efficient. Reductions in the paper work, safety improvement, data redundancy, data duplication and improved privacy and security are main features of EHR.

Benefits of EHR

Key benefits of using EHR to enable smart healthcare are listed below:

- **Effective maintenance of information**
  In EHR, data on paper is converted into soft form (as Excel files, database, etc.), and maintaining this data becomes easier and space effective. As data is in soft form, it can be stored more easily, and data retrieval becomes more efficient. Machine learning and data science tools and techniques can be applied on this data for drawing more insights and meaningful decisions. Healthcare organization can get more organized, sorted data on single click. Designing backup mechanism and policy formulation can also help to increase the lifetime of EHR.

- **Improved patient care**
  Generally, patients are treated by multiple healthcare service providers, and there is a need to exchange and sharing of information between them. As the EHR is stored centrally and maintained by trusted third-party IT service providers, this data can be available to healthcare organizations quickly. Past patient history, medical history of family, existing medications are readily available, and quick decisions can be taken to save patients life. Availability, reliability of data can help in reducing medical errors and better diagnosis.
- **Quality of care**
  EHR helps to improve quality of care by providing quick access to meta-data of the patient during observation, medication and treatment. It also enhances privacy and security of patient data giving patient assurance of their data. Due to soft data, billing time, waiting time is also reduced providing comfort to the patients. EHR also helps employees in healthcare organization to improve on productivity and work-life balance.
- **Cost optimization in service delivery**
  Ubiquitous services are integrated in smart healthcare applications which enable optimization in time and cost to deliver the services. Data aggregation and database federation mechanisms can also be associated with these services to provide the data across multiple healthcare organizations.
- **Improvement in research and best practices**
  As the data set from multiple healthcare organizations is available at central place, it creates better opportunities for researchers to initiate research on various medical problems solving using ICT. An interdisciplinary research can be initiated in a team of experts from various fields like medical expert, programmer, designer and data scientist. EHR also helps to establish ICT-based best practices to improve on the functioning of healthcare organization.
- **Improved safety**
  Through proper authorization mechanism, access control schemes and the policy of selective disclosure, the safety of EHR can be ensured. Through these solutions, patients can also be given more control on their personalized healthcare data.

EHR Implementation Issues

EHR always deals with data from various healthcare organizations and patients across the country, and its implementation in IoT and cloud environment is always critical issue. Designers have to design generic framework in order to deploy and implement EHR in any complex environment ensuring interoperability and backward as well as upward compatibility. The frameworks also need to mention the hardware and software requirements of platform on which EHR is going to be implemented. In addition to this, generic packages, interfaces also need to design to make them available readily to users, patients and healthcare organizations. The main factors which affect implementation of EHR are listed below [20]:

- **Dynamic clinical workflow**
  Operational and technical requirements of customers, patients as well as other stakeholders are continuously changing. This issue is very important while implementing EHR in any healthcare organization irrespective of the scale and other functional requirements. In the view of this, design of EHR should be in line with the policies and strategies of the healthcare organization. Implementation of EHR also needs significant changes in the dynamic workflow of the organization and is time-aware. Technical staff dealing with EHR, policy-makers, medical experts should also be taken into consideration and consulted while designing and implementing EHR for the organization.

- **Security issues**
  WHO has already declared EHR as most valuable assets of an individual than any other assets including money and other physical asset. Integrity and selective disclosure through authorized access to EHR is prime concern, and it should be addressed by adopting the emerging policy of security by design. As smart healthcare is integrated with IoT, there is a need of attack resistant security and privacy solution to ensure security and privacy of EHR to protect them from tampering and unauthorized access. Before deployment of security and privacy solution into the application, it is necessary to validate these solutions against known attacks to ensure that to what extent these solutions can fight against attacks. Essentially, in the context of EHR, prevention is more important instead of detection.

- **Naming and identification**
  Identity management while designing and implementing EHR in healthcare organization is very crucial issue. In fact, identity management itself is very big administrative domain and naming, unique identification, authentication, trust management are key functional components of this administrative domain. In smart healthcare application, patient's information in the form of EHR is collected through varied registration process using different identifiers, and when these EHR are aggregated at centralized location, unique identification of each EHR and its mapping to the respective healthcare organization from where it is collected is one of the import design issues. After centralized identity management system and federated identity management system, self-sovereignty [21] identity management solution is emerging in which decentralized identifiers [22] and verifiable credentials [23] are the main functional components. In self-sovereign identity management system, dynamic identity can be created with the help of distributed ledgers (i.e. blockchain [24]); however, an application of distributed ledger to the smart healthcare and IoT is still a debate.

- **Interoperability and compatibility**
  In smart healthcare applications, patient data in the form of EHR is collected from multiple healthcare organizations. The methods, APIs and functions which are used to aggregate EHR from multiple sources should be interoperable with each other. All healthcare applications are deployed on existing wired infrastructure, and the functionalities, services which are built on the top of these healthcare applications should be backward and upward compatible for the purpose of extending

these applications for scale or functional enhancements. Every smart healthcare application is designed and developed by different vendors with different assumptions, requirements and design issues. In the view of this, all methods, APIs and functions should be interoperable across variety of healthcare applications.

- **Standards**
  As mentioned earlier, interoperability and compatibility in both the ways are main design issues of EHR. In order to enable this across the globe, standardization is first and most important steps to bring uniformity in data formats, defining processes of collecting data across multiple healthcare organizations. Standards also bring global uniformity in clinical and business processes, data structure of EHR, maintaining QoS parameters of healthcare services and ensure security of EHR.

- **Operational complexity**
  Many employees in healthcare organizations dealing with healthcare organizations are not literate to use computers; therefore, they find it more time consuming to operate on the data due to lack sufficient knowledge of computer and their functionality. Special course material and training need to be designed and extended to such computer operators to reduce the operational complexity and experience the benefits of smart healthcare applications and EHRs.

2.5 Healthcare Projects

Government initiatives towards investments in smart city, smart country, advancement in ICT facilities, smart healthcare and E-Heath are increasing globally. More funds are being diverted to improve human life and prolong ageing. There are many successful projects in smart healthcare, and few potential projects are described below:

a. **Healthcare services to the patients with major depression (HELP4MOOD)**
   Depression is becoming the common problem among youngsters to old age people. It is one of serious problems causing social imbalance and increasing load on the healthcare organizations, government as well as caretakers. This project aims to provide self-guided treatment to the patients using computerized cognitive behavioural therapy [25]. Sensor movement, psychological ratings and voice analysis are monitored, and these details are provided to decision support system which is based on pattern recognition and machine learning. The potential outcomes of this project are smart monitoring, interactive system through virtual agents and intelligent decision support.

b. **MyHealthAvatar**
   Due to increasing patients across many chronic and non-chronic diseases, digitization of patient's details in the form of EHR is need of today. MyHealthAvatar [26] is one of the successful projects supported and funded by European Commission. Innovative medical care, volatile and long-term access to EHR, intelligent clinical decisions, personalized EHR to the patients and preventive measures are

the main objectives of this project. The main contribution of this project to the society is in enhancing the patient thought process, improvement in communication and updated search for the information balancing both social and economic fronts. It also opened many avenues to the industries and other stakeholders.

c. **Go-Smart**

Invasive treatment is becoming more popular in the view of patients across all age groups. Malignancy into and cancer is spreading at faster rate in human being and the main threat is that the cancer is passive for most of the time period and it is very difficult to detect whether the patient is suffering from cancer or not. Go-Smart [27] is one such project aims to provide smart minimally invasive cancer treatment to the patients by building open source software-based simulation platform which can support cancer. The data set generated from this simulation platform is also used by many researchers for analysis purpose in order to design preventive measures.

d. **iCARDEA**

Due to advancement in semiconductor industry and VLSI technology, use of BAN, especially cardiac implantable devices, has been growing exponentially. These cardiac implantable devices are resource constrained and small in size, and in the sequel, it needs software support in order to process data efficiently on the data centres. iCARDEA [28] is context-aware intelligent platform enabling proactive clinical guidelines which are very easy to interpret for medical experts. Personalized access to EHR through standard interfaces (e.g. HL7, ISO/IEEE 11073 and IHE IDCO) by ensuring security and privacy of the data is important feature of iCARDEA. In addition to these projects, readers can also look at other healthcare projects like closed-loop system for personalized and at-home rehabilitation of people with Parkinson's disease (CuPiD) [29], computer model derived indices for optimal patient-specific treatment selection and planning in heart failure (VP2HF) [30].

References

1. https://www.bccresearch.com/market-research/healthcare/preventive-healthcaretechnologies-hlc070a.html.
2. https://www.expresshealthcare.in/eh-budget-2020/healthcare-budget-2020/416703/.
3. Shinde, G. R., Kalamkar, A. B., Mahalle, P. N., et al. (2020). Forecasting Models for Coronavirus Disease (COVID-19): A Survey of the State-of-the-Art. SN COMPUT. SCI.
4. www.bcbs.com.
5. FIESTA-IoT, www.fiesta-iot.edu.
6. Durga, S., Nag, R., & Daniel, E. (2019). Survey on machine learning and deep learning algorithms used in internet of things (IoT) healthcare. In *3rd International Conference on Computing Methodologies and Communication (ICCMC)*.
7. Contractor, D., & Telang, A. (2017). *Applications of cognitive computing systems and IBM Watson*. Springer.

8. Salehi, S. A., Razzaque, A., Tomeo-Reyes, I., & Hussain, N. (2016). IEEE 802.15.6 standard in wireless body area networks from a healthcare point of view. In *Proceedings of the 22nd Asia-Pacific Conference on Communications (APCC)*, Yogyakarta (pp. 523–528).
9. Ghamari, M., Janko, B., Sherratt, R. S., Harwin, W., Piechockic, R., & Soltanpur, C. (2016). A survey on wireless body area networks for ehealthcare systems in residential environments. *Sensors, 16*(6), 831.
10. Shinde, G. R. (2017). Cluster framework for internet of people, things and services. Ph.D. Thesis, Aalborg University.
11. Movassaghi, S., Abolhasan, M., Lipman, J., Smith, D., & Jamalipour, A. (2014). Wireless body area networks: a survey. *IEEE Communication Surveys & Tutorials, 16*(3), 1658–1686.
12. Hardt, D. (2012). The OAuth 2.0 authorization framework.
13. Seitz, L., Selander, G., Wahlstroem, E., Erdtman, S., & Tschofenig, H. (2018). Authentication and authorization for constrained environments (ACE) using the OAuth 2.0 framework (ACE-OAuth). IETF, Internet-Draft draft-ietf-ace-oauth-authz-11.
14. Maler, E., Catalano, D., Machulak, M., & Hardjono, T. (2016). User-managed access (UMA) profile of OAuth 2.0.
15. Protecting Personal Data in a IoT Network with UMA [Online]. Available: https://www.slideshare.net/kantarainitiative/uma-auth-ziotirmdublinv06. Accessed 9 May 2017.
16. Mahalle, P. N., Sable, N. P., Mahalle, N. P., & Shinde, G. R. (2020). Data analytics: COVID-19 prediction using multimodal data. In A. Joshi, N. Dey, K. Santosh (Eds.), *Intelligent systems and methods to combat Covid-19*. SpringerBriefs in Applied Sciences and Technology. Springer, Singapore.
17. McDuff, D. J., Estepp, J. R., Piasecki, A. M., & Blackford, E. B. (2015). A survey of remote optical photo plethysmographic imaging methods. In *2015 37th Annual International Conference of the IEEE Engineering in Medicine and Biology Society (EMBC)* (pp. 6398–6404).
18. Chen, M., et al. (2014). A survey of recent developments in home M2M networks. *IEEE Communications Surveys & Tutorials, 16*(1), 98–114.
19. Mainanwal, V., Gupta, M., & Upadhayay, S. K. (2015). A survey on wireless body area network: security technology and its design methodology issue. In *2015 International Conference on Innovations in Information, Embedded and Communication Systems (ICIIECS)* (pp. 1–5).
20. Sinha, P., Sunder, G., Bendale, P., Mantri, M., & Dande, A. (2012). *Electronic health record: standards, coding systems, frameworks, and infrastructures*. Wiley. https://doi.org/10.1002/9781118479612. Print ISBN: 9781118281345, Online ISBN: 9781118479612.
21. Allen, C. (2016). The path to self-sovereign identity. Life With Alacrity.
22. Reed, D., Sprony, M., Longley, D., Allen, C., Grant, R., & Sabadello, M. (2018). Decentralized Identifiers (DIDs) v0. 11 Data Model and Syntaxes for Decentralized Identifiers (DIDs). W3C.
23. Sporny, M., Burnett, D. C., Longley, D., & Kellogg, G. (2018). Verifiable credentials data model 1.0–expressing verifiable information on the web. Draft, 7.
24. Mahalle, P., Shinde, G., & Shafi, P. (2020). Rethinking decentralised identifiers and verifiable credentials for the internet of things. In *Internet of things, smart computing and technology: A roadmap ahead* (pp.361–374). Springer.
25. https://cordis.europa.eu/project/id/248765.
26. https://cordis.europa.eu/project/id/600929.
27. https://cordis.europa.eu/project/id/600641.
28. https://cordis.europa.eu/project/id/248240.
29. https://cordis.europa.eu/project/id/288516.
30. https://cordis.europa.eu/project/id/611823.

Chapter 3
Big Data, Healthcare and IoT

3.1 Introduction to Big Data

"Big data refers to the tools, processes and procedures allowing an organization to create, manipulate, and manage very large data sets and storage facilities"—according to zdnet.com.

As per Gartner's definition [Circa 2001]: Big data is defined in 3 Vs. Data that contains greater variety in growing volumes and with ever higher velocity.

The data is coming from different sources with more complex data sets in structured, semi-structured and unstructured format. Hence, there is need of processing this large amount of data to perform business centric analysis. Big data creates challenges in data extraction, transfer, encryption, storage, indexing, analysis and visualization.

Big data has a complex nature that requires powerful technologies and advanced algorithms. So, the traditional business intelligence tools can no longer be efficient in the case of big data applications [1].

As shown in Fig. 3.1 the data available in large amount with different sources and type is known as big data.

The data is coming in different scale, sources, types and forms. These are well describing the four Vs namely volume, velocity, variety and veracity. Big data made drastic change in the Web 2.O company strategies. The research became more focussed on handling larger data, contribution towards open source technology that changed the concerted software development, scale and hardware infrastructure economics.

A data scientist will be skilful at managing volume and by building algorithms to make intelligent use of the size of the data as efficiently as possible.

Volume: Big data exceeds the capacity of traditional databases. The amount of data generated every day is near about 2.5 quintillion bytes of data due to the growth of Internet of things (IoT). So, the data is interactive form which contains the browser

© The Author(s), under exclusive license to Springer Nature Singapore Pte Ltd. 2021
P. N. Mahalle and S. S. Sonawane, *Foundations of Data Science Based Healthcare Internet of Things*, SpringerBriefs in Computational Intelligence,
https://doi.org/10.1007/978-981-33-6460-8_3

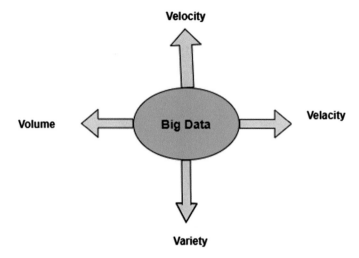

Fig. 3.1 Big data

activity, sensors data, RFID data, digital recorder, phone, etc. The analysis deals with finding the correlation between data elements.

Velocity: The data velocity is accelerating. The data stream of tweets, posts, financial information is coming from many users in increasing way. The velocity increases data volume exponentially. Instagram is good example of that illustrates the impressive growth of data. Over 700 million people use the Instagram.

Variety: As the computing power is increased, data available is more than 100 features. Big data comes from various heterogenous sources in structured or unstructured form.

Veracity: Veracity deals with certainty and consistency of big data [2]. Veracity is positively associated with volume, velocity and variety of data.

The change in variety, velocity and volume demands new metrics and tools.

Along with these Vs, additional Vs and other characteristics [3] are used to better define big data: Vision (a purpose), Verification (processed data to deal with some specifications), Validation (the fulfilled purpose), Value (relevant information can be extracted for many sectors), Complexity (difficulty in organizing and analysing big data because of evolving data relationships) and Immutability (collected and stored big data can be permanent if well managed).

3.2 Healthcare Challenges

Eminence healthcare [4] is one of the most important issues in how individuals perceive their quality of life. As per WHO guidelines (www.un.org), next 10 years would be decade of action to deliver the global goal into three levels of

1. Global action: More resources and greater leadership for sustainable development goals.
2. Local action: Embedding the needed transitions in the policies, budgets, institutional framework of governments, cities and local authorities.
3. People action: Civil society, youths, academia to generate movement pushing the required transformation.

Reasons of growing complexity of Healthcare data

1. New technologies [5] are developed in order to

   a. Mobile applications
   b. Sensors
   c. Capturing devices.

2. More incentive to medical professionals to use electronics health records.
3. Social network is playing important role in communication, searching the medical-related information.
4. More medical knowledge is being collected.

3.3 Big Data Challenge in Healthcare

Health data is increasing day by day at a huge scale, at various levels of phenotyping [1] and from different types of resources. Addressing the latent and challenges of big data in healthcare requires an understanding of the characteristics of the data.

Based on the characteristics and importance of various features of healthcare data, the qualitative big amount of data is used for analysis. Table 3.1 shows the characteristics of healthcare data. The table shows the various characteristics and their respective data records. The data comes from different sources, domains and states.

The healthcare data is associated with the difference properties based on its basic structure, correlation and sources which are shown in Table 3.2.

Table 3.1 Characteristics of healthcare data

S. No.	Name of characteristics	Description
1	Sources	Electronic health record, patients self-records, Internet, biobanks [6], clinical registries
2	Domain	Administrative health data, biomarker data, biometric data and imaging
3	States	Structured versus unstructured, patient care-oriented versus research-oriented explicit versus implicit (for example, check-up's versus social media) raw versus ascertained (data without processing versus data after standardization and validation processes)

Table 3.2 Data properties of healthcare data

S. No.	Data property	Description
1	Sample size	
2	Phenotyping depth	Persons genome and biological derivatives Demographic factors Lifestyle habits Clinical phenotyping Psychological phenotyping Environmental phenotyping
3	Data correlation	Associative between subjects
4	Standardization of data	Through collaboration among countries
5	Linkage between data sources	Using common ID across all the sources to understand common pattern and provide suitable treatment and a way to become data accessible, interoperable and reusable

Types of healthcare data sources [7]

1. Electronic Health Records: It includes patient's medical history in the digital form.
   Examples: Problems, medications, physician's observations, medical history, laboratory data radiology reports, progress notes, billing information.
2. Biomedical Image: Medical imaging plays very important role in the analysis due to high-quality images of anatomical structure in human beings.
   Examples: magnetic resonance imaging (MRI), computed tomography (CT), positron emission tomography (PET) and ultrasound (U/S).
3. Sensor Data: Used majorly for real-time data and retrospective analysis.
   Data collection units for examples: electrocardiogram (ECG) and electroencephalogram (EEG).
4. Clinical Data: It is in the form of clinical notes and in the unstructured form. This contains clinical information in the form from transcription of dictation and speech recognition process.
5. Social Media Data: There is rapid growth in social media resources such as Websites, blogs/microblog, chatbots, discussion forums and online communication which provides the views about public opinion on different aspects of healthcare.

Large amount of medical data has significance to identify the association, classification, diagnosis and treatment and behaviour of disease. Major step includes here is creating an accurate predictive model describing all mentioned tasks (Fig. 3.2).

1. Clinical note in unstructured and semi-structured format is necessary to understand in the right context and analyse it.
2. The patient's data is coming from various sources hence inferring knowledge from heterogenous patient sources and finding the association/correlation between longitudinal records.

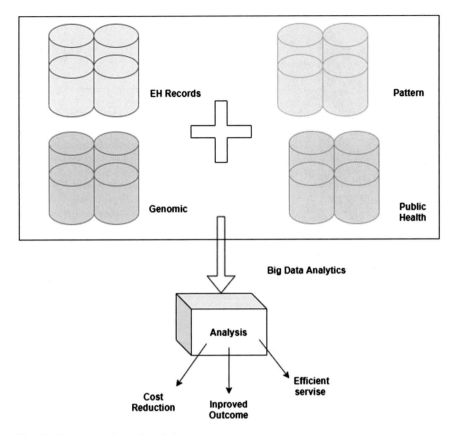

Fig. 3.2 Big data analytics: broad view

3. The medical imaging data is available in large amount, hence extracting pattern efficiently.
4. Genomic data analysis.
5. Combining genomic and clinical data analysis.
6. Study and capture patient's behavioural data through different types of sensors.

3.4 Data Science for Healthcare IoT

Data science has been defined into three distinct ways of analysis tasks: description, prediction and counterfactual prediction. These tasks can be defined and used as described in Fig. 3.3.

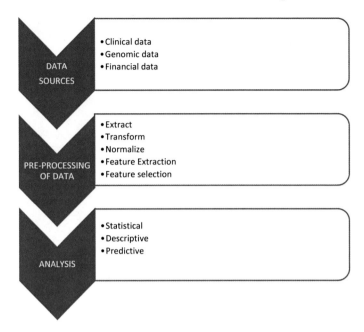

Fig. 3.3 Process of analysis of data

In the process of data analysis, the data is extracted from relevant source and cleaned, normalized and transformed using data pre-processing methods. The relevant features are selected using feature selection method. The dimensions of data are reduced in the step of feature extraction.

Descriptive analysis

Descriptive analysis is finding association between features in order to provide a quantifiable summary of certain features.

For example: Finding BMI over time in children. Descriptive analysis methods are important to find exploratory study of the data and extract interesting patterns of the data.

Prediction analysis

Prediction analysis is learning an association between a set of inputs to some outcome of interest, such that it can afterword be used to predict the outcome from the inputs in a different unseen set. It is thus applied in settings in which there is a well-defined task. Prediction analysis holds the potential for improving disease diagnostic and prognostic.

Few examples of predictive analysis in healthcare include assisting medical treatment by capturing patient's behaviour and interactions and analysis of diagnosis.

Medical big data ability depends on the extraction of meaningful information from large-scale resources in order to improve the understanding of human health. Medical data is transformed into following broad categories

1. Disease diagnosis, prevention.
2. Modelling disease progression.
3. Genetic impact.
4. Environmental influence.
5. Improving the health process.

3.5 Text Analytics in Healthcare

Because of the advances in clinical field, the data is majorly available in the form of text documents. Appropriate analysis of document helps physician, hospitals and expert to improve the quality of care service, finding the best appropriate treatments. A personalized, predictive and effective medicine can be approached by incorporating advanced techniques.

The basic importance of text mining methods in the field of healthcare is discussed here.

1. **Name Entity Recognition**: A named entity is defined as a word that identified its class for example a person, a place, an organization, a date or time and quantity. In the healthcare system, NER is mainly used to extract concept as well as term.

   a. **Medical concept**: Extraction of medical concepts like drug, injury and disease in the clinical text.
   b. **Time expression**: The accurate extraction of time expressions in the medical field like date of onset of a disease, duration and frequency of the treatment is a really important.
   c. **Personal data anonymization**: The protection of personal data has become a challenge for many health institutions, especially with the rising computerization of almost any clinical record.
   d. **Relation extraction**: The discovery of semantic relationships, e.g. connections among diseases and symptoms, between medical concepts is essential. The relation like disease-treatment, disease-test, and disease-symptom is essential to identify.

2. **Text summarization**: Summarization method is used to identify the main topics of a document and create a summary which includes its key points. This is therefore a really important technique that allows the important information to be read by healthcare professionals in a reduced substantial time.

   a. Extractive method [8, 9]: These methods can be defined as a discovery of significant sentences from the text document that represents the summary. PERSIVAL(PErsonalized Retrieval and Summarization of Images, Video and Language), extractive and multidocument summarization system is a framework that performs a different summary strategy depending on the type of user (physician or non-professionals).

    b. Abstractive method [10]: The information is presented by constructing new contents and analysing meaning of the original text. SemRep is tool representing the useful relation between the text elements. (https://skr3.nlm.nih.gov/SemMed/), a Web application based on the SemRep system and the UMLS Metathesaurus that automatically summarizes all the MEDLINE citations returned by a PubMed search. Semantic MEDLINE provides four types of summaries: diagnosis, substance interaction, treatment of a disease and pharmacogenomics. One of its major features is the resulting summarization, which is shown in the form of a graph to ease its clarity.

3. **Text Classification** [11]: Nowadays, automatic text classification has become an essential task in medicine especially due to the quantity of textual information available in many disparate sources (databases, articles, social networks, forums, news, etc.).

    a. **Automatic diagnostic classification**: The task of classifying medical reports written in natural language by finding diagnostics into 52,000 codes of International classification of diseases version 10 (ICD10).

    b. **Patient stratification**: It is a process of classifying certain clinical characteristics of patients from free-text radiological reports. Authors presented a multiclass classification system to automatically identify smoking status (current smoker, past smoker, past or current smoker, non-smoker and unknown status) from unstructured electronic health records.

    c. **Medical Literature Classification**: It is a task of classifying medical literature from the MEDLINE database.

Tools

1. MEDLINE [2] and PubMed Database[12]:

    a. It is the U.S. National Library of Medicine® (NLM) premier bibliographic database.

    b. It contains more than 26 million references to journal articles in life sciences focussed on biomedicine.

    c. A distinguishing feature of MEDLINE is that the records are indexed with NLM Medical Subject Headings (MeSH®).

    d. PubMed is information retrieval system which gives access to MEDLINE documents.

2. **UMLS Project** [13]:

    a. The Unified Medical Language System (UMLS) project is a long-term National Library of Medicine research and development effort

    b. It is designed to provide the retrieval and integration of information from multiple machine-readable biomedical information sources.

    c. It has three components Metathesaurus, the Semantic Network and the SPECIALIST Lexicon.

    d. This is mainly used for NLP application in the application of healthcare

3. **Data set**

    a. GENIA (https://www.nactem.ac.uk/genia).

    b. ONCOTERM (https://www.ugr.es/~oncoterm/) complete repository of information about the complex terminology associated with cancer.

    c. NCBI disease corpus (https://www.ncbi.nlm.nih.gov/CBBresearch/Dogan/DISEASE/) is a relevant annotated corpus used to perform TM tasks, e.g. disease named entity recognition.

4. **Ontologies**

    a. Disease Ontology (DO) (https://disease-ontology.org/). It is an open source ontology consisting of 8,043 hereditary, developmental and acquired human diseases.

    b. GALEN (https://bioportal.bioontology.org/ontologies/GALEN), an open ontology that includes anatomical concepts, diseases, symptoms, drugs and procedures, as well as the existing relationships between entities. Fi

5. **Thesaurus:**

    a. Unified Medical Language System (UMLS) (https://www.nlm.nih.gov/research/umls) is a repository of multiple controlled vocabularies (more than 150) in biomedical sciences and healthcare.

    b. Medical Subject Headings (MeSH) (https://www.ncbi.nlm.nih.gov/mesh) is a controlled vocabulary thesaurus for indexing and classifying biomedical and health-related information.

    c. Systematized Nomenclature of Medicine Clinical Terms (SNOMED-CT) (https://www.snomed.org/snomed-ct) is a multilingual clinical healthcare terminology that includes three types of component: concepts, descriptions and relationships.

6. **Advanced text pre-processing and analysis tools:**

    a. MetaMap (https://metamap.nlm.nih.gov/), a widely used tool in medicine whose main aim is to get relevant concepts in a wide collection of biomedical texts by using as terminological and semantical basis the UMLS Metathesaurus.

    b. Apache cTAKES (clinical Text Analysis and Knowledge Extraction System) (https://ctakes.apache.org/) is an open source system specifically designed for the extraction of relevant information from electronic medical records.

References

1. Shilo, S., Rossman, H., & Segal, E. (2020). Axes of a revolution: Challenges and promises of big data in healthcare. *Nature Medicine, 26*(1), 29–38.
2. https://www.nlm.nih.gov/bsd/medline.html.
3. Emani, C. K., Cullot, N., & Nicolle, C. (2015). Understandable big data: A survey. *Computer Science Review, 17,* 70–81.
4. Mora, H., et al. (2017). An IoT-based computational framework for healthcare monitoring in mobile environments. *Sensors, 17*(10), 2302.
5. Dang, L. M., et al. (2019). A survey on internet of things and cloud computing for healthcare. *Electronics, 8*(7), 768.
6. Organization for Economic Cooperation and Development. (2006). Glossary of statistical Terms: biobank. In: *Creation and Governance of Human Genetic Research Databases (OECD).* https://stats.oecd.org/glossary/detail.asp?ID=7220.
7. Wang, L., & Alexander, C. A. (2019). Big data analytics in healthcare systems. *International Journal of Mathematical, Engineering and Management Sciences, 4*(1), 17–26.
8. Joshi, S. G., & Sonawane, S. S. (2015). A survey of extractive summarization approaches using graph model. *International Journal of Computer Engineering and Applications, 9*(4), 145–156.
9. Sarwadnya, V. V., & Sonawane, S. S. (2018). Extractive summarizer construction techniques: A survey.
10. Moratanch, N., & Chitrakala, S. (2016, March). A survey on abstractive text summarization. In *2016 International Conference on Circuit, power and computing technologies (ICCPCT)* (pp. 1–7). IEEE.
11. Kowsari, K., Jafari Meimandi, K., Heidarysafa, M., Mendu, S., Barnes, L., & Brown, D. (2019). Text classification algorithms: A survey. *Information, 10*(4), 150.
12. https://pubmed.ncbi.nlm.nih.gov/.
13. Nelson, S. J., Powell, T., & Humphreys, B. L. (2002). The Unified Medical Language System (UMLS) project. In: Encyclopedia of Library and Information Science.

Chapter 4
Data Science Techniques, Tools and Algorithms

4.1 Introduction

We live in the world where data is everywhere. Websites, Smartphone records your interest, location, profile and perform update at every second. There are smart gazettes which are recording your heart beats, moving pattern, sleep data and diet information. Extensive knowledge is available in this huge data, and extraction is the study of data science.

LinkedIn network asks you to list the current job and location so as to recommend the user of the same profile and increase the network. It also analyses the people working in the company similar to your profile and provides job recommendation.

The famous Indian premier league, which is a famous twenty-twenty cricket league, performs the analysis of data in depth. The best bowler and batsman, the top performer, the best team, the team lost the greatest number of matches, role of winning toss in the victory and many more analysis can be performed on the data.

As per Joseph E. Gonzalez, data science definition is the application of data-centric, computational and inferential thinking to understand the world and solve problems.

Data science is a process of extracting knowledge from data.

Data science [1] not only is a synthetic concept to unify statistics, data analysis and their related methods but also comprises its results. It includes three phases, design for data, collection of data and analysis on data.

Machine learning is used to extract knowledge and make decision-making intelligent.

There are broad two methods:

Supervised learning methods

In supervised learning, a system produces decisions/outputs based on input data. Spam filters and automated credit card approval systems are examples of this type of learning.

P. N. Mahalle and S. S. Sonawane, *Foundations of Data Science Based Healthcare Internet of Things*, SpringerBriefs in Computational Intelligence,
https://doi.org/10.1007/978-981-33-6460-8_4

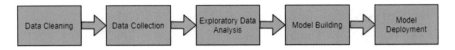

Fig. 4.1 Data science process

Unsupervised learning methods

Unsupervised learning is a process of rearranging the inputs in order to organize an unlabelled data. A good example is clustering, which takes a collection of elements, each with a number of features, and partitions the entity space into sets or groups based on nearness of the attributes of all elements.

Data Science Process: The data science process is described in Fig. 4.1.

Data Cleaning: The cleaning is an important step of the process. If your data is clean, you can proceed to construct good model.

Model Building: It is the analysis of data to create a model that best fits the data.

Model Deployment: It presents your findings.

4.2 Data Science Techniques

In this section, the important techniques of data science are introduced in detail.

4.2.1 Classification

The data classification [2] has huge applications. As the relationship between different attributes with class variables is available, the problem is specified as

> Given a set of training data values along with associated labels, determine the class label for an unlabelled test example.

Classification algorithms typically contain two phases:

1. Training Phase: In this phase, a model is constructed from the training examples.
2. Testing Phase: In this phase, the created model is used to assign a label to an unlabelled test example.

In this section, the different methods that are commonly used for data classification will be discussed in brief.

Attribute types

1. **Discrete**: Data takes certain values, e.g. number of students in the class.
2. **Categorical**: Take data within the range, e.g. time.

4.2.1.1 Feature Selection Methods

In the data collection phase, the data collected contains wide number of attributes. The irrelevant attributed may generate poor model. Hence, it is important to use the correct features during the training phase. There are broad two types:

1. Filter Models: The algorithm to extract suitable feature or subset of features is applied in order to find their suitability for classification. To perform feature selection models, a number of measures are used in order to quantify the importance of a feature for classification process.
2. Wrapper Model: The classification method includes feature selection method [3] so as to make it sensitive to the classification process. At each iteration, the classification algorithm evaluates a particular set of features. This set of features is added as per greedy strategy and tested to see the quality improves. This approach generates a feature set which is sensitive to the classification algorithm.

Measures used for feature selection using filter models are given as below:

Let $p_1 \ldots p_k$ be the fraction of classes that corresponds to a particular value of the discrete attribute.

1. Gini Index: The Gini index of that value of the discrete attribute is given by:

$$G = \sum_{i=0}^{k} p_i^2$$

The value of G ranges between 0 and $1 - 1/k$. The overall Gini index for the attribute can be measured by weighted averaging over different values of the discrete attribute or by using the maximum Gini index over any of the different discrete values.

2. Entropy: The entropy of a particular value of the discrete attribute is measured as follows:

$$E = \sum_{i=1}^{k} p_i \cdot \log(p_i)$$

The value of the entropy lies between 0 and $\log(k)$.

3. **Chi-square**: When the class variable is categorical, this test is used to select the feature.

$$(X)^2 = \sum_{i=1}^{n} \frac{(O_i - E_i)^2}{E_i}$$

$(X)^2$ is the summation of the squared difference between observed and expected frequencies divided by the expected frequency for all the cells.

4. **Fisher Index**: The Fisher index [4] measures the ratio of class scatter to within class scatter. p_j is the fraction of training examples of class j, and μ_j is the mean of particular feature for class j. μ is the global mean for that feature, and σ_j is the standard deviation of that feature for class j. Fisher score is computed as

$$x = \frac{\sum_{i=1}^{k} p_j \cdot (\mu_j - \mu)^2}{\sum_{i=1}^{k} p_j \cdot \sigma_j^2}$$

4.2.1.2 Decision Tree

Decision trees perform a hierarchical partitioning of the data, which relates the different partitions at the leaf level to the different classes. The partitioning at each level is created with the use of a split criterion. The split criterion may be either on a single attribute or on multiple attributes. The overall approach is to try to recursively split the training data so as to maximize the discrimination among the different classes over different nodes. The discrimination among the different classes is maximized, when the level of skew among the different classes in a given node is maximized. Gini index or entropy is used to select the attributes for splitting.

The Gini index and entropy provide an effective way to evaluate the quality of attribute selection.

Training: Split the data recursively. The terminating condition is one where all data records belong to the same class.

Testing: The new data is tested on the constructed decision tree to find the class label.

The decision tree is pruned in order to handle overfitting. There are generally two methods to prune the tree:

1. Minimum description length principle in deciding when to prune a node from the tree.
2. Hold out a small percentage of the training data during the decision tree growth phase. It is then tested to see whether replacing a subtree with a single node improves the classification accuracy on the hold-out data set. If it happens, then the pruning is performed.

In the testing phase, a test instance is assigned to an appropriate path in the decision tree, based on the evaluation of the split criteria in a hierarchical decision process. The class label of the corresponding leaf node is reported as the relevant one.

4.2.1.3 Rule-Based Method

Rule-based methods are similar to decision trees, but they do not have splitting data set. Any path in the decision tree is example of rule. The set of disjoint rules are possible to create from the different paths in the decision tree. Rule-based classifiers are general model. There are chances of getting overlapping of rule with the existing one. It works in two phases.

Training Phase: The rules are extracted from the training data.

Testing Phase: The rules are identified which match to the test example. The class labels are extracted and combined to get the final result.

Many times, the target class labels are different for a particular test example. To handle this case, the rule sets are checked for ordered and unordered case. If the rule sets are ordered, then the top matching rules are used to get the prediction of classes. While if it is unordered, then the voting is used by the rules to make the prediction.

RIPPER [5] is rule-based system which works in two stages:

The first stage is a greedy process which constructs an initial rule set.

The second stage is an optimization phase which attempts to further improve the density and accuracy of the rule set.

The algorithm is extended to use for text categorization problem. The Boolean feature is identified for each word appearing in the corpus. If the word is available, it is set as true for the corresponding document. A corpus of n documents by m words are used and represented by $n * m$ matrix. Accordingly, the rules are constructed. The test document is iterated over the features and generates an attribute, and the class is predicted.

4.2.1.4 Probability-Based Method

The most basic method for classification is probability-based methods. The statistical inferences are used to find the best class for a given example.

Prior probability: Fraction of training records belonging to each class.

Posterior probability: Probability of observing the specific characteristics of the test instance.

The probabilistic classifier predicts the posterior probability of test example. There are two standard cases to estimate the posterior probability.

1. By applying Bayes theorem.
2. Learn the discriminative function to map input feature vector to class label.

Bayes Theorem: It is the most known method of generative model. Consider a test example with different features, which have values $X = x_1 \dots x_l$, respectively. To find the posterior probability that the class $Y(T)$ of the test instance T is i, we need to find the posterior probability

$$P(Y(T)) = i|x_1 \dots x_l).$$

Then, the Bayes rule can be used in order to derive the following:

$$P(Y(T)) = \frac{P(x_1, x_2, x_3, \dots x_d)|Y(T) = i)}{p(x_1, x_2, x_3, \dots x_d)}$$

Denominator is constant across all classes, so the expression becomes as follows:

$$P(Y(T)) = P(x_1, x_2, x_3, \ldots x_d)|Y(T) = i)$$

The above expression can be expressed as the product of the feature-wise conditional probabilities.

$$P(x_1, x_2, x_3, \ldots x_d|Y(T) = i) = \prod_{j=1}^{l} P(x_j|Y(T) = i)$$

This equation is referred as conditional independence. The term is computed as multiplication of feature values x_j for the jth attribute where the training data corresponds to ith class. If the particular data is not available, i.e. for zero probability problem, the Laplacian smoothing technique is applied in order to estimate the values robustly.

The Bayes rule is successful in wide number of applications and very popular in text classification as well.

Another probability-based method is to directly model posterior probability. Discriminative function learns to map the input feature vector to class label. The approach is called as discriminative model. Logical regression is discriminative classifier. It is determined by using the following equation

$$P(Y(T)) = \frac{1}{1 + e^{-\theta^T X}}$$

The maximum likelihood is used to estimate the vector of parameter θ. The logistic regression model is used in many applications like Web and medical field.

4.2.1.5   SVM Classifiers

Binary classification problem is well handled using support vector machine. The class label y_i for the ith training instance X_i is assumed to draw from $\{-1, +1\}$. It is called as maximum margin hyperplane.

4.2.1.6   Instance-Based Learning

The test examples are directly related to training examples in order to create a classification model. It is also called as lazy learning methods. Nearest neighbour method is an example of instance-based leaning. The top k-nearest neighbours are identified for the test example. The class label occurring maximum time among k-nearest neighbours is reported as the relevant class label. Many variations are available for instance-based learning. It is based on the reduction of noise in the clustering phase and use of appropriate similarity method for accurate results.

4.2.1.7 Semi-supervised Learning

The additional labelled or unlabelled data is used to improve the performance of classification algorithm. Semi-supervised learning methods improve the effectiveness of learning methods with the use of unlabelled data, when only a small amount of labelled data is available. Transfer learning is the method where the external labelled data is used. In case of semi-supervised learning, unlabelled data with the same feature is used. The unlabelled data provides density structures in terms of clusters and sparse regions. The feature correlations and joint feature distributions are helpful for classification.

The motivation behind using semi-supervised learning is that knowledge of correlated regions of the space and dense regions for classification.

The two-class problem is shown in Fig. 4.2a using normal classification and using unsupervised learning for data classification. It shows the impact of unsupervised learning as the sample margin is shifted as the training instances of unlabelled data. The correlation between variables is estimated, and joint feature distribution can be estimated with unlabelled data.

For example, consider the case where the training data is available to predict whether the given document is in the "COVID-19" category. There may be a case where the word "examination" may not occur in any of the training documents. However, the word "examination" may be available with "COVID-19" category in the unlabelled examples. Thus, the unlabelled examples can be used to learn the less common features for the classification process in case when the data is small.

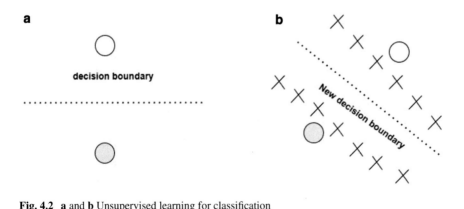

Fig. 4.2 a and **b** Unsupervised learning for classification

When the clustering is applied, each cluster in the data contains data record of one class. Hence, cluster label provides critical information to its classification process. In many of the domains, the addition of unlabelled data provides significant advantages for the classification process.

4.2.1.8   Ensemble Learning

It is a meta-algorithm which reuses one or more existing classification algorithm by combining the results. The aim of the algorithm is to find accurate results from multiple training model.

The error in the classification model depends on the bias and variance.

Bias: Bias is the difference between average predicted value and actual value which we are trying to predict.

Variance: Variance is the variability of model prediction for a given data point or a value which tells us spread of our data.

1. Boosting: Create models to classify the data points in different portions of the data set. Then, it combines scores over all the components. Applying different classifiers and combining the result work well on all parts of the data.
2. Bagging: Training examples are chosen randomly by sampling with replacement. The results are combined from the models constructed using different samples.
3. Random Forest: Random forests are a method which uses set of decision trees. It uses bagging when building a decision tree. It combines together result to make accurate prediction.
4. Stacking: Combination of classifier is performed in stacking. The out-of-different first-level classifiers are used in second-level classifier, and the first-level classifier may use bagging method and different classifiers. To avoid overfitting, the training data needs to divide into two subsets for first-level and second-level classifier.
5. Model averaging: Bayesian methods are used to combine the model. The error caused due to bias of particular classifier is handled by using different classifiers.

4.2.2   Cluster Analysis Methods

Clustering is a process of forming a cluster/group of similar data objects. The data objects in a cluster are similar to each other, while the data objects in different clusters are not related to each other.

It is an unsupervised technique where the class labels are not available with the examples.

The following are the different types of clustering.

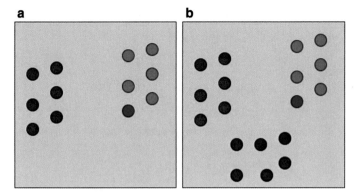

Fig. 4.3 **a** Two clusters and **b** three clusters

4.2.2.1 Clustering Types

1. Partitional: Partitional method is the method of separating data objects into non-overlapping subsets. Figure 4.3a, b shows collections of partitioned clusters.
2. Hierarchical: The clusters have subclusters in this type. The nested clusters form a tree. Every intermediate node is union of its subclusters. The leaf nodes represent data objects.
3. Exclusive: The data object is assigned to single cluster. No data objects are placed in more than one cluster. While in non-exclusive type data, object can belong to more than one cluster.
4. Fuzzy: The membership weight is of a data object calculated between 0 and 1. The membership with the cluster is represented with weight. Here, addition of weight of each object is always 1. The weight represents its association with the cluster.
5. Complete: In this type, the category of the cluster is defined, whereas in the partial clustering type some objects may not belong to the well-defined groups.

4.2.2.2 Clustering Techniques

In this section, three important clustering techniques are introduced: K-means, agglomerative and DBSCAN.

Similarity Computation

Accurate clustering requires a precise similarity between pairs of data objects. Different similarity or closeness or distance measures [6] have been proposed and widely used. Some of the measures are discussed in this section.

1. Euclidean distance: Euclidean distance is widely used method in clustering. D_1 and D_2 are the document vectors. The distance of the data objects is calculated as

$$\text{Dis}(D_1, D_2) = \sum_{i=1}^{n}(D_{1i} - D_{2i})^2$$

2. Cosine Similarity: It is the cosine angle between the vectors of two documents.

$$\text{COS}(D_1, D_2) = \frac{D_1 \cdot D_2}{\|D_1\| \|D_2\|}$$

Cosine is the angle between two vectors D_1 and D_2 of size n. $\|D_1\| = \sqrt{D_{11}^2 + D_{12}^2 + D_{13}^2 + \cdots + D_{1n}^2}$.

3. Jaccard Coefficient: Jaccard metric measures the similarity as the intersection divided by the union of data objects. The measure is

$$\text{JSIM}(D_1, D_2) = \frac{D_1.D_2}{|D_1|^2 + |D_2|^2 - D_1.D_2}$$

The Jaccard coefficient is 0 when both the vectors are disjoint and 1 when D_1 and D_2 are same.

4. Pearson Correlation Coefficient: It is another measure to find the extent of which two vectors are related. General form of the coefficient is as follows:

$$\text{PSIM}(D_1, D_2) = \frac{m \sum_{t=1}^{m} w_{t,a} \times w_{t,b} - \text{TF}_a \times \text{TF}_b}{\sqrt{\left[m \sum_{t=1}^{m} w_{t,a}^2 - \text{TF}_a^2\right].\left[m \sum_{t=1}^{m} w_{t,b}^2 - \text{TF}_b^2\right]}}$$

where $\text{TF}_a = \sum_{t=1}^{m} w_{t,a}$ and $\text{TF}_b = \sum_{t=1}^{m} w_{t,b}$. This measure ranges from $+1$ to -1, and it is 1 when both document vectors are same.

K-Means Algorithm

It is prototype-based clustering where data objects in a cluster are more similar to the prototype which defines the cluster than any other cluster. The prototype may define as mean/average or medoid of all the points in the cluster.

It is a partitional clustering method based on value k which is represented by its centroids.

The basic algorithm is as follows:

1. K value is taken from user which is number of clusters. K initial centroid is considered.
2. Each point is assigned to a centroid of cluster.

3. The centroid is refined according to the point assigned to the cluster.
4. The assignment and updating centroid repeated until no change in cluster or until centroid remains same.

Here, the distance between data points with the centroid is calculated at each iteration. K-means is also used for document data. Document data is represented as term document matrix. Important point is to increase the similarity of the document in the cluster to the cluster centroid. Cluster cohesion is used which is given below

$$\text{Total Cohesion} = \sum_{i=1}^{K} \sum_{x \in C_i} \text{cosine}(x, c_i)$$

where x is an object, K is number of clusters and C_i is the ith cluster.

Though K-means is simple and used for different data types, it is not used for all types of data.

Also, it failed to handle clusters of different sizes. The main issue with K-means algorithm is null cluster may get formed if no points are allocated to a cluster during the assignment phase. Also, when outliers are there in the data, cluster centroid is not good representative. Finally, K-means is restricted to the data for which a notion of a centroid is defined.

Agglomerative Hierarchical Clustering

Hierarchical clustering techniques are another important type of clustering method. There are two basic techniques for generating a hierarchical clustering:

1. Agglomerative: It starts with the data points as individual clusters. The closest pair of clusters are merged as per the proximity measure.
2. Divisive: It starts with one all-inclusive cluster. Later split the cluster until only singleton clusters of individual points remain. In this case, we need to decide which cluster to split at each step and how to do the splitting.

In this section, we will focus exclusively on agglomerative hierarchical clustering method. A hierarchical clustering is often displayed graphically using a tree-like structure called a dendrogram, which displays both the cluster–subcluster relationships and the order in which the clusters were merged (agglomerative view) or split (divisive view). The sample dendrogram is shown in Fig. 4.4.

Basic algorithm is as follows:

1. Compute the similarity between the data objects of clusters. Cluster similarity is computed using techniques like MIN, MAX, AVERAGE. MIN defines cluster similarity to the closest data points between two different clusters. MAX provides similarity between the farthest data points between two different clusters. AVERAGE is the average of all pairs of data point from different clusters.
2. Merge the closest clusters.

Fig. 4.4 A sample of
four-point clustering using
dendrogram

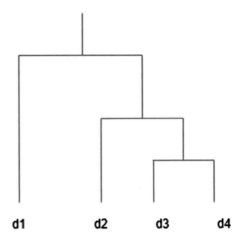

3.   Perform steps 1 and 2 until one cluster left.

As this technique decides the objective function locally at each step, it avoids the difficulty of attempting to solve a hard combinatorial optimization problem. It also has advantage of taking different cluster sizes into account.

However, agglomerative hierarchical clustering algorithms tend to make good local decisions about combining two clusters since they can use information about the pairwise similarity of all points. However, once a decision is made to merge two clusters, it cannot be undone at a later time.

The clusters generated are better quality, but method is computational and storage point expensive.

DBSCAN

DBSCAN is density-based clustering algorithm which is simple and effective.

In the centre-based approach, density is estimated for a particular point in the data set by counting the number of points within a specified radius of that point. This includes the point itself.

The centre-based approach to density classifies a point as being

(1)   In the interior of a dense region (a core point): These points are in the interior of a density-based cluster. A point is a core point if the number of points within a given neighbourhood around the point is determined by the distance function and a user-specified distance parameter.
(2)   On the edge of a dense region (a border point): It falls within the neighbourhood of a core point.
(3)   In a sparsely occupied region (a noise or background point): It is neither a core point or a border point.

The algorithm is as follows:

1. Label given points as core, border or noise points.
2. Discard the noise points.
3. Put an edge between all core points within radius of each other.
4. Make a cluster of core points.
5. Assign each border points to one of the clusters.

Because DBSCAN uses a density-based definition of a cluster, it is relatively resistant to noise and can handle clusters of arbitrary shapes and sizes. Thus, DBSCAN can find many clusters that could not be found using K-means.

However, DBSCAN has trouble when the clusters have widely varying densities. It also has trouble with high-dimensional data because density is more difficult to define such data.

Finally, DBSCAN can be expensive when the computation of nearest neighbours requires computing all pairwise proximities, as is usually the case for high-dimensional data.

4.2.3 Regression

Regression is a statistical technique to find the relationship between variables. Linear regression is a powerful technique for analysing data. In linear regression, data is fit in a line $y = \beta_0 + \beta_1 x$. X is called independent, and y is response variable. β_1 is slope of a line, and β_0 is the intercept of a line. The paired data points are observed, and we assume that y_i is generated by using line that we evaluate at $x_i \cdot \varepsilon$ is the noise in the data.

$$y = \beta_0 + \beta_1 x + \varepsilon$$

Multiple linear regression or multivariate regression used vector and matrices to represent the equation

$$Y = X\beta + \varepsilon$$

Deep Learning

At the core of deep learning are neural networks: mathematical entities capable of representing complicated functions through a composition of simpler functions.

Neural network term provides a link to the way our brain works. Both artificial and physiological neural networks use vaguely similar mathematical strategies for approximating complicated functions because that family of strategies works very effectively.

The basic building block is neuron which I denoted by the following

$$o = f(wx + b)$$

o is output, w and b are learned parameter, x is input, and f is activation function.

In general, x, w, b and, hence, o can be simple scalars or vector-valued (meaning holding many scalar values) and similarly, w.

This expression is referred to as a layer of neurons, since it represents many neurons via the multidimensional weights and biases.

A multilayer neural network, as represented in following equation, is made up of a composition of functions.

$$O = f(w_n(\ldots F(w_2(f(w_1 * x + b_1) + b_2)) + \cdots + b_n)$$
$$X_1 = f(w_0 * x + b_0)$$
$$X_2 = f(w_1 * x_1 + b_1)$$
$$\ldots$$
$$Y = f(w_n * x_n + b_n)$$

where the output of a layer of neurons is used as an input for the next layer. w_0 here is a matrix, and x is a vector. Using a vector allows w_0 to hold an entire layer of neurons, not just a single weight.

The main difference between linear model and model for deep learning is error function shape. Our linear model and error-squared loss function had a convex error curve with a singular, clearly defined minimum. Neural networks have non-convex error surfaces due to the activation function. The ability of an ensemble of neurons to approximate a very wide range of useful functions depends on the combination of the linear and nonlinear behaviour inherent to each neuron.

The activation function is important in inner parts of the model which allow to have different slopes to output function at different values, and at the last layer of the network it has the role of concentrating the outputs of the preceding linear operations into a given range.

Deep neural networks give us the ability to approximate highly nonlinear phenomena without having an explicit model for them. Instead, starting from a generic, untrained model, it is a task by providing it with a set of inputs and outputs and a loss function from which to backpropagate.

4.3   Cognitive Healthcare IoT

The integration of cognitive computing in IoT devices is nowadays in great demand. The thought process of human is simulated using the computerized model. In 2020, there are more hat 29 billion devices connected to IoT network. Cognitive IoT refers to the infusion of logical reasoning and thinking capabilities to the data which is collected by IoT devices.

In case of healthcare domain, it has become essential to get the accurate and faster analysis.

There are three phases of cognition:

1. Understanding: Understand the large volume of data structured or unstructured and derive meaning from it.
2. Reasoning: Use the model to derive the answers.
3. Learning: Automatically infer the new knowledge from data.

The reason behind using cognitive computing for IoT devices is

(a) Data generation scale and rate.
(b) Characterize the intelligent behaviour of objects.
(c) Integration of multiple data types and sources.

The simple case is of patient who is admitted in the hospital monitored through sensor-enabled devices. Cognitive IoT learns the data of patients who are monitored in the same siltation earlier and triggers the alarm of notification to doctors and patients based on the situation of patients.

Cognitive IoT(CIoT) [7] is advancing field which is used to create tremendous applications to improve health care. The remote monitoring of patients, tracking, generation of alert, medical equipment control and many more elements are in cognitive IoT. Rapid response and medical emergencies can improve using CIoT. It connects sensors on patients' body and monitors health data and persons' physiological signals.

All data objects like sensor and devices are interconnected to understand the physical and social environments, and it stores and processes the learned information and the extracted knowledge and learns to adapt themselves. It minimizes hum intervention by making intelligent decision processing system.

Cognitive IoT smart healthcare scenario is proposed by Alhussein et al. [7] to access electronic health records as shown in Fig. 4.5.

In the proposed smart healthcare monitoring framework, different types of health-related multimedia and EEG signals are obtained using smart IoT sensors. The network transmits the signals from IoT devices to computing devices. These smart devices transmit received data to the cloud via wide area network layer.

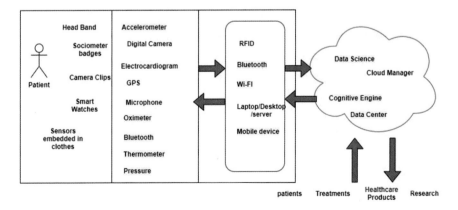

Fig. 4.5 Cognitive IoT smart healthcare scenario [7]

The cloud has the cloud manager, data centre, data science server. The cloud manager authenticates whether a resident is registered with a smart healthcare provider. The cloud manager is also responsible for verifying the identity of all stakeholders in the smart healthcare system, such as doctors, medical staff members, hospital representatives and patients. The cloud manager also controls the data flow to and from the various servers and manages communication, storage and other resources. The cloud manager sends the data to the cognitive engine, which uses multimodal data including EEG and psychological and physiological data and determines whether the patient needs emergency care. The sensor signals also include patient's movements, gestures, facial expressions to know about the patient's state. The cognitive system then makes a real-time decision based on patient's state, about the activities and the medical attention, services to be provided to the patient and whether to send data to the deep learning module.

4.4 Case Studies: Frameworks and Projects

In this section, two case studies related to NLP applications are explained.

4.4.1 CASE STUDY #1: Text Summarization of Medical Documents

Here, text summarization of biomedical document is proposed by Mozhgan Nasr Azadani et al. [2] as case study. This method makes use of Unified Medical Language System (UMLS) [8] to construct a concept-based method. The concepts of sentences are identified, and similarity is computed between the sentences which is represented using graph. The best related sentences are extracted by applying graph clustering method. Finally, the sentences which describe the theme of document are extracted as summary.

Text summarization is divided into two types:

1. Extractive Summarization [9–12]: Extract important sentences from the document and putting them together in a summary.
2. Abstractive Summarization: Extract the meaning of text and produce the summary using language generation tools. It required paraphrasing of sentences.
3. Hybrid Approach: Perform extractive summarization and extract useful sentences and later apply extractive summarization to get theme of document in summary.

Motivation

Information overload in the health sector is becoming an important problem which is necessary to address [13]. The data is available in clinical notes [14], guidelines and scientific literature. Less time, heavy workload and resources may cause problems such as mistakes, inefficiency, communication failures.

It is also applicable in reducing biomedical paper by preserving most significant points.

Also, mostly the biomedical texts have important characteristics like variety of acronym, synonyms, abbreviations and hypernyms. For example, the words like stroke and cerebrovascular accidents are related to brain illness. A concept-based analysis of medical document is necessary to find the related terms together to generate the summary of document.

Graph [15] is represented for document where node is lexical or semantic unit like concept, term, sentences, paragraphs, phrase and relation is similarity between two node elements. The similarity relation is weighted. Ranking algorithm is applied to find the important nodes, and summary is extracted.

The similarity between the nodes is computed using cosine similarity method, common subsequence or using TextRank [16] model. These methods do not take into account domain-specific knowledge.

Method

This method uses graph-based system to generate extractive summarization. In this method, data mining method frequent itemset mining is used to extract the concepts from the document. It takes into account the similarity between sentences using concept. Later, the most scored and related sentences are extracted to generate the summary (Fig. 4.6).

1. Text Processing

The pre-processing steps are needed to remove the unwanted elements from the text document. The elements which are not necessary are removed in this module. The input text is divided into tokens. Stop words are removed from the text. The stemming is applied, and noun groups are formed. The extra pre-processing like removing figures/diagrams or tables is removed from the summary. The short forms and special words are handled in this section.

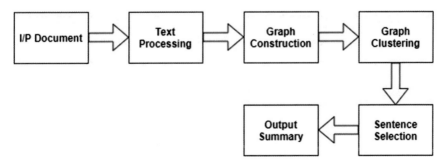

Fig. 4.6 Architecture

Concepts are extracted using UMLS. There are three important sources.

(1) Metathesaurus: It consists of biomedical concepts with its synonym
(2) Semantic Network: The semantic categories with semantic relation of Metathe-
    saurus.
(3) Specialist Lexicon: Extensive lexicon used in NLP system.

The biomedical concepts are discovered using MetaMap tool. It is used to map
the biomedical concept to the UMLS Metathesaurus. The text sentences and noun
phrases are extracted from each sentence. The MetaMap tool generates all candidate
concepts mapped to specific noun phrase. It returns the concept with higher score. It
uses the entire vocabulary set to return the related concepts.

Example (1): Sentence ID and sentences

The following are the sentences:

1. "Psychiatric disorders are common in the population and result in considerable
   morbidity and mortality."
2. "Over the decades, psychiatric classification systems such as the Diagnostic and
   Statistical Manual of Mental Disorders and the International Classification of
   Diseases."

To provide the appropriate data format, frequent itemset mining is used. Transaction set is used as data format. It has transaction ID and items field. Each document
consists of set of sentences. In the previous step, the concepts are extracted. These
concepts are used to represent each sentence in the transaction set.

Example (2): Concepts extracted of sentences given in example 1

1. Mental disorders, abnormal behaviour, population group, experimental result.
2. Psychiatric classifications, togo, tryptophanase, diagnosis, oprelvekin, reporting,
   inform, therapeutic procedure, administration procedure, biomaterial, treatment,
   treatment epoch, treatment–act information management reason, professional
   guide, research.

2. **Graph Construction**

The weighted graph is constructed using transactional data format created in the
previous section. Vertices are the sentences, and edges are similarity between these
sentences. The correlation between these concepts is calculated using frequent
itemset mining. The set of items which occurs frequently are identified as frequent
itemset. The frequent itemset covers a transaction if it includes all items in the transaction. Support of itemset is calculated by taking ratio of number of transactions it
covers by the total transaction.

Finally, the itemset is considered as frequent if it is greater than the minimum
support value.

After finding the frequent k-itemset, these are used to represent a given document. Similarity between two sentences is carried out by Jaccard coefficient. The

Fig. 4.7 Graph construction

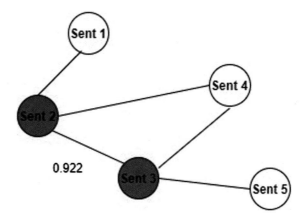

intersection of frequent items is divided by the total items. Hence, the similarity is nothing but the semantic content overlap between two sentences of a given sentence (Fig. 4.7).

3. **Graph Clustering**: the sentences having more common frequent itemset that convey more semantic and meaning are identified using this step

This cluster aims to find the sentences which cover related themes of document in the final summary. Minimum spanning tree-based clustering algorithm is used to find the cluster. The more similar sentences are put in cluster, while the sentences which are different are in another cluster.

Each sentence with max values is assigned in new cluster. If one of the sentences has been already clustered, then new unattached sentence is added to this cluster.

Figure 4.8 shows the sample three clusters generated using algorithm. The sentences within a cluster are more related than the sentences outside the cluster.

4. **Sentence Selection**

The sentences are selected from the generated clusters. The sentence selection strategy depends on the common frequent subsets and hence provides theme of the document. It also covers subtheme of document; hence, redundancy is avoided.

Finally, summary sentences are selected from each cluster based on the ranking on their similarity measure. The top scorer sentences are chosen. Hence, each cluster has a role in generating the summary.

The selected sentences appear in the final summary based on their original order in the given document so as to maintain the order.

The system can adequately resolve the intrinsic ambiguities of biomedical literature in comparison with traditional term-based methods and select the most informative sentences using clustering approach. Also, the standard metric ROUGH is used for analysis purpose which has been shown that the proposed summarizer outperforms another keyword-based, statistical feature-based or term frequency summarization systems.

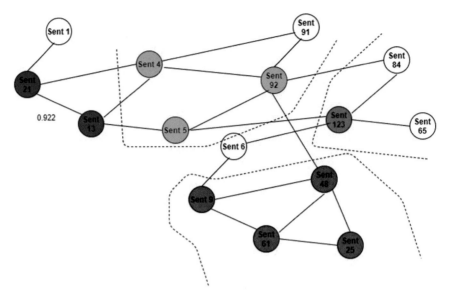

Fig. 4.8 Graph clustering

Hence, the single document biomedical text summarization is proposed in this case study, while the integration of difference knowledge sources may improve the performance of the system.

4.4.2 CASE STUDY #2: Automatic Summarization Methods for Clinical Free Text Notes

This case study is the discussion of the research paper by Hans Moen et al. [17].

The original discharge summary is typically written by a physician. These summaries are generally extracted from accompanying clinical notes. These notes are generally follow-up treatment information.

Data

The clinical note is unstructured. Sample text is given in Fig. 4.9. There is no standardized structure to write clinical note. These are normally applied at the end of the patient's hospital stay or after they are discharged from hospital.

61-years old female with Crohn's disease. Attended cycling event in Salo, flu priror1ry. Arfter cycling, experienced breathing difficulties and went to the emergency department and elevated herart enzymes and incompensation were found. Was admitted to the ICU for care of incompensation and pneumonia. In UKG 2.6. ef 30%. In coronary angiography, significrant stenoses in RCA, LCX and mrarin. Trordray, elective quadrurple bypass LITA-LAD, Ao-LOM-LPL and Ao-RBD, in which goord flow. Pre.op. the posterior wall of the left ventricle and the septum contract lamely, ef about 35%, mitral valve 1-2/4 leak. Aortic cross-clamp time 1 h 32 min. Post.op. ef over 40%. On basis of the UKG-finding pre.op. Simdax-infusion was initiated. On arrival to ICU, haemodynamics was stable, norepinephrine administered. Cardiac index 3,2. Warming-up and weaning in ventilator.

Fig. 4.9 Sample clinical note [17]

Method

1. Repeated Sentences Method

As per the observation in the clinical notes, most of the information is repeated. Repeated sentences [18] method is used to generate the summary. The idea is that the point written in multiple notes is the most important information to add to the summary. The features from initial sentence scoring are used, and the order score is added to generate the final score. The highest scoring sentences are included in the final summary. The repeated sentences summarization method is illustrated in Fig. 4.10.

Post-processing is applied to each summary to arrange the sentence order. It is sorted according to the date of clinical note written.

2. Case-Based Summarization

It uses case-based reasoning (CBR). The most similar case care episode (as per clinical notes) has similar content in their discharge summaries. These summaries are used to extract theme/topic. The sentences with these topics are extracted, and similar sentences are mined using cosine similarity measure. The higher score sentences are included in the summary.

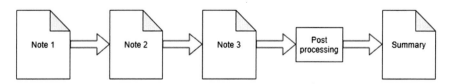

Fig. 4.10 Multidocument summarization of clinical notes

The following four steps are applied:

1. Retrieve top 5 episodes.
2. Score sentences in the query by computing similarity to each sentence by retrieving episode discharge summary.
3. Use the generated summary to write the final discharge summary.
4. Store the new summary in electronic health record for further use.

The above steps are used as base-based cycle in the hospital to avoid the inefficiency and redundancy.

This case study provides useful directions on how to approach this summarization task in a resource-lean fashion. Further studies are required to assess the applicability of such methods in real-world clinical settings [19, 20].

4.5 Economic Growth

Manyika et al. [10] estimate a potential economic impact from IoT of $3,900–$11,100 billion per annum (pa) in 2025. This is leading to growing numbers of machines and devices connected to the Internet. As per Manyika et al. [10], IoT will contribute 4 to 11 per cent of total world GDP in year 2025. IoT will be going to impact both consumers and industries. Chinese cellular IoT connections accounted for 15% of world connections in 2010, and 61% in 2018. The IOT connections for the US are 28% in 2010 and 11% in 2018 (Fig. 4.11). According to [9], the Chinese large-scale adoption of IoT has been driven by investments in connected cars, smart metering, payment terminals, industrial applications and smart cameras.

As per the work carried by Zainab Alansar et al., these results provide an important insight of IoT in healthcare domain in economic success by 45.32% and to the quality of life by 31.05%. As per the researchers and experts, the weight of environmental

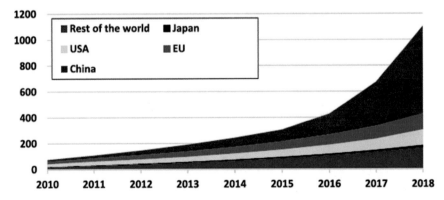

Fig. 4.11 Number of IoT connections in the world [9] as per GSMA wireless intelligence database (2019)

protection to develop IoT smart health sector is 23.63%. Therefore, it is recommended to the policy-makers of the health sector to focus on developing the new technologies such as IoT application on economic criteria like employment and revenue, then social criteria such as increasing the welfare of patients and citizens and satisfaction of hospital personnel in the use of medical tools.

References

1. Hayashi, C. (1998). "What is data science? Fundamental concepts and a heuristic example." *Data science, classification, and related methods* (pp. 40-51). Springer, Tokyo.
2. Agrawal, C. C. (2014). *Data classification algorithms and applications.* CRC Press.
3. Liu, H., & Motoda, H. (2012). *Feature selection for knowledge discovery and data mining.* (Vol 454). Springer Science & Business Media.
4. Gu, Q., Li, Z., & Han, J. (2012). Generalized fisher score for feature selection. *arXiv preprint* arXiv:1202.3725.
5. Cohen, W. W., & Singer, Y. (1999). Context-sensitive learning methods for text categorization. *ACM Transactions on Information Systems (TOIS), 17*(2), 141–173.
6. Huang, A. Similarity measures for text document clustering. In *Proceedings of the Sixth New Zealand Computer Science Research Student Conference (NZCSRSC2008)* (Vol. 4), Christchurch, New Zealand.
7. Alhussein, M., et al. (2018). Cognitive IoT-Cloud Integration for Smart Healthcare: Case Study for Epileptic Seizure Detection and Monitoring. *Mobile Networks and Applications* 23(6), 1624–1635.
8. Nelson, S. J., Powell, T., & Humphreys, B. L. (2002). The Unified Medical Language System (UMLS) project. In: *Encyclopedia of Library and Information Science.*
9. Edquist, H., Goodridge, P., & Haskel, J. (2019). The Internet of Things and economic growth in a panel of countries. *Economics of Innovation and New Technology*, 1–22.
10. Manyika, J., Chui, M., Bisson, P., Woetzel, J., Bughin, J., & Aharon, D. (2015). *The internet of things: mapping the value beyond the hype.* San Francisco: McKinsey Global Institute.
11. Sonawane, S., Kulkarni, P., Deshpande, C., & Athawale, B. (2019). Extractive summarization using semigraph (ESSg). *Evolving Systems, 10*(3), 409–424.
12. Sonawane, S., Ghotkar, A., & Hinge, S. (2019). Context-based multi-document summarization. In *Contemporary advances in innovative and applicable information technology* (pp. 153–165). Singapore: Springer.
13. Hall, A., & Walton, G. (2004). Information overload within the health care system: A literature review. *Health Information & Libraries Journal, 21*(2), 102–108. https://doi.org/10.1111/j.1471-1842.2004.00506.x.
14. Van Vleck, T. T., Stein, D. M., Stetson, P. D., & Johnson, S. B. (2007). Assessing data relevance for automated generation of a clinical summary. In J. M. Teich, J. Suermondt, & G. Hripcsak (Eds.), *AMIA Annual Symposium Proceedings* (pp. 761–765).
15. Azadani, M. N., Ghadiri, N., & Davoodijam, E. (2018). Graph-based biomedical text summarization: An itemset mining and sentence clustering approach. *Journal of biomedical informatics*, 84, 42–58.
16. Mihalcea, R., & Tarau, P. (2004). TextRank: Bringing order into text. In *Proceedings of the 2004 Conference on Empirical Methods in Natural Language Processing* (pp. 404–411).
17. Moen, H., Peltonen, L. M., Heimonen, J., Airola, A., Pahikkala, T., Salakoski, T., & Salanterä, S. (2016). Comparison of automatic summarisation methods for clinical free text notes. *Artificial intelligence in medicine*, 67, 25-37.
18. Meng, F., Taira, R. K., Bui, A. A., Kangarloo, H., & Churchill, B. M. (2005). Automatic generation of repeated patient information for tailoring clinical notes. *International Journal of Medical Informatics, 74*(7–8), 663–673.

19. Lissauer, T., Paterson, C., Simons, A., & Beard, R. (1991). Evaluation of computer-generated neonatal discharge summaries. *Archives of Disease in Childhood, 66*(4 Spec No.), 433–436.
20. SumPubMed: Summarization Dataset of PubMed Scientific Articleshttps://vgupta123.github.io/docs/sumpubmed_mainpaper.pdf.

Chapter 5
Conclusion

This section concludes the book and proposes the future outlook which can be explored further to initiate new research avenues.

5.1 Open Research Issues

Advancement in BAN and biomedical sensors has made healthcare applications more ubiquitous in nature. However, use of IoT devices in healthcare domain is creating many open research problems. Healthcare data is very critical, and there is a need to exchange this data from devices to middleware at faster rate. In the sequel, delay-aware data exchange requires faster and lightweight algorithms to run at both the sides. Optimization in performance metrics like energy consumption, packet delivery ratio, end-to-end delay and throughput is open problem and requires more efficient algorithm to optimize these parameters. Reliability of IoT devices for capturing physiological parameter is very important issue, and the role of material science is very critical and important. Data storage of big volume is one of the important challenges in healthcare domain. Many healthcare organizations prefer to store this data at the local server. However, due to increasing volume the local servers are not adequate and there is a need to integrate IoT with cloud. Nowadays, cloud-based storage based on IT infrastructure is being adapted by healthcare organizations. Cloud service providers also offer guaranteed security as well as economical solutions, and legal service level agreement is also signed by service providers. Better techniques and algorithms need to be researched further for IoT cloud convergence. Efficient data management and drawing of meaningful insights require complete and live meta-data of stored data. Meta-data includes timestamp, owner of the data, location, access details. This meta-data is useful for the version management and to data analyst as well as researchers. Design of better techniques and mechanisms for fetching this meta-data is another open research problem. Querying also becomes more easy and

P. N. Mahalle and S. S. Sonawane, *Foundations of Data Science Based Healthcare Internet of Things*, SpringerBriefs in Computational Intelligence, https://doi.org/10.1007/978-981-33-6460-8_5

efficient due to availability of meta-data to draw more meaningful insights. Design of accurate query tools and their interoperability with the data set is an interesting area to research further.

As the healthcare data is very critical and can lead to human deaths, accuracy and security are very important issues. There are many studies available in the literature [1, 2] which shows that aggregation of patient clinical data into EHR is not accurate always. The possible reasons for this are the lack of knowledge, poor EHR system design, inaccurate workflows in RPM, etc. Discrepancy management mechanism plays very important role in maintaining the accuracy of this clinical data, and it can be also improved by observing the flaws in workflows. Security of EHR and related clinical data is of prime concern. There are various possible attacks on EHR which includes attack on identity, integrity, denial of service attack and emerging ransomware as well as phishing attack. Threat analysis and vulnerability analysis are required to design attack-resistant security solution for the healthcare domain. Formulating security guidelines and security assessment framework also require more research.

Research in medical and healthcare domain is dependent on the availability of sufficient time series data set of the patients. There has been lot of research in data analytics of pandemic like COVID-19 [3, 4] and similar other diseases. Several imaging techniques used in healthcare domain are computed tomography, magnetic resonance imaging, X-ray, ultrasound imaging, and all requires strong image analytics. Images captured in these techniques are high resolution and large in size, and designing more accurate data science algorithms and techniques is an important research area.

More than 80% of clinical data is available in unstructured format; hence, there is heavy need of performing to apply advanced skills to analyse this type of data. Patients' health data, physician notes, IoT collected data, electronics medical records, insurance providers, social media data and Web knowledge are the important data sources of healthcare data. Most of these sources are in unstructured format. Researchers and experts are using text analytics model and natural language processing to analyse data from these sources. The following are some of the advantages of using natural language processing in health care:

1. Cost reduction in administrative process by facilitating fast billing process, extracting relevant information from clinical notes to avoid delay in further process.
2. Efficient decision support system by predicting post-surgical complications and streamlining assessment of medical policy.

The NLP techniques and model are successful in faster detection of changes in the clinical reports and guidelines, extract named entities (concepts) from EHR for identification of diseases and developing automation of machine-assisted surgery guided by human instruction.

A recent study using text analytics and sentiment analysis in mental health looked at suicidal ideation. NLP promises to push the healthcare industry forward by providing sophisticated use of NLP to enable patients and professional to use rich data sources and improving the quality and efficiency of healthcare delivery.

5.2 Future Outlook

There are many issues and challenges related to data science and IoT healthcare integration which have not been considered in the scope of this book. There are several opportunities and research avenues which can be explored and built on the top of contents presented in this book. This section presents these possibilities and open issues for future research.

As there is minimum human intervention in IoT healthcare applications, resource-constrained IoT devices are always engaged in processing. However, we will require some delegation mechanism for faster and accurate insights from the big data. In addition to this, better decision support, customized and personalized healthcare information for an individual, complex prediction, integration of cutting-edge tools, model overfitting in decision support software can be also important areas to explore further.

In healthcare applications, the clinical data is collected across diverse and heterogeneous platforms and data scientist has bigger challenge to integrate and implement solutions for this. There is a need of new tools and technologies to address nature, complexity and velocity of this clinical data. Data science in healthcare domain also can be linked to drug discovery organization and come up with more effective drugs by studying the life cycle of clinical data since inception.

Data science is used to advance health and reduce disparities [5] from data to information, information to knowledge and from knowledge to evidence-based practice. Health disparities require the interaction of influences at various levels at individual, family, community and social over the life course, the variety of relevant mediator and the interacting mechanism available. Big data science is changing the medical practices and public health scenario. Health data has different axes which represents different properties. Analysis of big data in health aims at providing wider perspective on states of health and disease.

Predictive analysis' main objective is to alert health professional of the likelihood of events and outcomes before they occur. It helps them to prevent as much as cure health issues. As IoT use is increasing day by day, the algorithms have not only historical but also real-time data. Predictive data science helps to support clinical decision at the individual level as well as applicable to hospitals' operational and administrative challenges.

Text analytics is helping healthcare industry to create a personalized recommendation, understand high-risk patients and improve the outcome. It can be useful not in the today's problem but also be expanded to solve future use cases.

Data science tools [6] can also be used for contact tracing of the COVID-19 case to identify hotspots and to alert people. The healthcare industry is changing as the delivery models are changing. Cognitive health care has ability to scale expertise and help organizations to use their own data effectively for predicting the knowledge. There is heavy need of healthcare industry to prepare own path towards becoming a cognitive industry.

References

1. Valikodath, N. G., et al. (2017). Agreement of ocular symptom reporting between patient-reported outcomes and medical records. *JAMA Ophthalmology, 135*(3), 225–231.
2. Echaiz, J. F., et al. (2015). Low correlation between self-report and medical record documentation of urinary tract infection symptoms. *American Journal of Infection Control, 43*(9), 983–986.
3. Shinde, G., Kalamkar, A., Mahalle, P., & Dey, N. (2020). *Data analytics for pandemics.* Boca Raton: CRC Press. https://doi.org/10.1201/9781003095415.
4. Bhapkar, H. R., Mahalle, P. N., & Dhotre, P. S. (2020) Virus graph and COVID-19 pandemic: A graph theory approach. In A. E. Hassanien, N. Dey, S. Elghamrawy (Eds.), *Big data analytics and artificial intelligence against COVID-19: Innovation vision and approach. studies in big data* (Vol. 78). Springer.
5. Zhang, X., Pérez-Stable, E. J., Bourne, P. E., Peprah, E., Duru, O. K., Breen, N., et al. (2017). Big data science: Opportunities and challenges to address minority health and health disparities in the 21st century. *Ethnicity & Disease, 27*(2), 95.
6. Review of Big Data Analytics, Artificial Intelligence and Nature-Inspired Computing Models towards Accurate Detection of COVID-19 Pandemic Cases and Contact Tracing.

Printed in the United States
By Bookmasters